Muscle Energy Techniques

A Practical Guide for Physical Therapists

JOHN GIBBONS

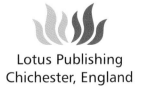

Lotus Publishing
Chichester, England

First published in 2011 by
Lotus Publishing
Apple Tree Cottage, Inlands Road, Nutbourne, Chichester, PO18 8RJ and

Drawings Amanda Williams
Photographs Ian Taylor
Text and Cover Design Wendy Craig
Printed and Bound in the UK by Scotprint

MEDICAL DISCLAIMER: The following information is intended for general information purposes only. Individuals should always see their health care provider before administering any suggestions made in this book. Any application of the material set forth in the following pages is at the reader's discretion and is his or her sole responsibility.

British Library Cataloguing-in-Publication Data
A CIP record for this book is available from the British Library
ISBN 978 1 905367 23 8

Name
Comment
Author's signature

Contents

Preface

I have been lecturing in the field of physical therapy for many years and am sometimes disappointed that I meet many students who have been taught *muscle energy techniques* (METs) but do not really have an understanding of what they are all about.

If I were honest I would say with hand on heart that I use an MET, or a variation of one, with every patient whom I treat, and I feel it is a major component of the overall treatment plan. Without METs I would still have success with my patients' symptoms, but when I incorporate an MET I feel that it is 'the icing on the cake' in enabling my patients to experience a reduction of their symptoms.

I wanted to write a book so that the subject of METs could not only be easily understood by a student of physical therapy, but also be useful to the qualified physical therapist. This book should appeal to anybody in the physical therapy field who would like to have easy access to METs without overcomplicating the subject.

Even on my five-year osteopathy programme, *muscle energy techniques* were a very small component of the course, and I was very disappointed with the way in which the whole subject of METs was covered, to the point that my fellow students did not understand when and how an MET is used.

From that day onwards I vowed that I would write a book in a very simple and straightforward way so that every student – whether of osteopathy, chiropractic, physiotherapy or sports massage therapy – would be able to understand METs and, more importantly, be able to apply them to their patients without any confusion.

Acknowledgements

I feel very honoured and extremely privileged to be able to produce this book through Jon Hutchings of Lotus Publishing. As you can imagine, like most books, it has taken many painstaking hours to put together; and finally it is done.

I must thank Robert White of Physique Management, who is also my best friend – without his involvement, this book would never have been published. I also want to say that Robert has been like a father figure to me over the years, as well as a good friend; he has helped me on numerous occasions to pursue my dream within my physical therapy career – thanks again.

I would like to say something about my son, Thomas Rhys Gibbons: he is eleven at the moment as I write this book. I hope that he will achieve great things in his life and that I will be an inspiration to him as he is to me. Part of the writing of this book was for you, Tom – I wanted to show you that, with self-motivation and, more importantly, having a goal in your life, anything can be achieved. I have really enjoyed the last eleven years being your father and I hope you have enjoyed your time with me. I will always be there for you and I love you so very much – you will always be known as Tom-Tom to me.

I lost my father to cancer when I was only nine years old – I hope I am around for my son for many more years to come. Part of my drive to progress and be successful in my life is the fact that I didn't have a father figure in my teenage years. I wanted to follow in my father's footsteps and join the forces, so I enrolled in the army when I was sixteen years old. I still think of you every day, Dad, and I miss you so very much.

To my mother, Margaret Gibbons, and my sister, Amanda Williams – I want to thank you with all my heart for putting up with me when I was a troublesome teenager. This book is to demonstrate that, with determination and persistence, something can be achieved in a person's life even if they underachieve in school.

Someone else I would like to mention and thank is Norman Basson. Norman was an ex-military physiotherapist who taught me sports therapy many years ago. I found him to be a great tutor of physical therapy and I feel that he gave me the inspiration to pursue my dream. Without Norman's mentoring and guidance, this book would not have been possible.

I would like to mention and thank Leon Chaitow for all the books that he has produced over the years for osteopaths and physical therapists. His books have allowed therapists to gain a better understanding of physical therapy, whether they are an osteopath, chiropractor, physiotherapist or physical therapist. Leon, I can only aspire to what you have achieved in your life, and I hope you will find my book of interest.

My thanks go to one of the models, Jack Meeks, of the University of Oxford Sports Department.

And, finally, to Denise, my fiancé and future wife – thank you. Denise was the main model in the book and the greatest of supporters, allowing me the freedom to achieve my dreams.

Anatomical Terminology

1

The anatomical position provides a standard reference point for an individual: the body is upright, with the head, eyes and toes all facing forwards, and the arms and hands are hanging by the sides, palms turned to the front.

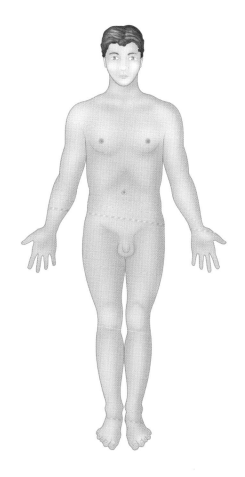

Terms to Describe Position and Direction

Afferent   Directed inwards to an organ or a part of the body, e.g. spinal cord.

Anterior   Situated at or towards the front of the body. Also called ventral. A term prefixed with antero signifies 'before'.

Deep   Situated far away from the body surface.

Distal   Remote or away from any point of origin of a structure. From Latin distans, meaning 'distant'.

Dorsum   The back or posterior surface of something, e.g. back of the hand, or upper surface of the foot.

Efferent   Directed away from an organ or a part of the body.

Inferior   Situated below, or directed down, away from the head. Also known as caudal.

Lateral   Towards the side, or located away from the midline, of the body or organ.

Medial   Towards the midline of the body or organ.

Palmar   Relating to the anterior surface (palm) of the hand.

Peripheral   Towards the outer surface of the body or organ.

Plantar   Relating to the posterior surface (sole) of the foot.

Posterior   Situated at or towards the back of the body. Also called dorsal. Postero is a combining form, denoting a relationship to the posterior part, e.g. posterolateral.

Prone   Position of the body in which the ventral (anterior) surface faces down.

Proximal   Nearest or closer to any point of origin of a structure. From Latin proximus, meaning 'next'.

Superficial   Situated near or at the body surface.

Superior   Situated above, towards the head. Also known as cephalic.

Supine   Position of the body in which the ventral (anterior) surface faces up.

Other Terms

Agonists   Muscles that provide most of the force required for movement. Also known as prime movers.

Antagonists   The opposing muscle group of the agonists.

Contracture   Refers to the degree of shortness that results in a marked loss of range of motion.

Muscle imbalance   A condition that exists when a muscle is tight and strong and its antagonist is generally lengthened and weakened.

Shortness   Refers to a degree of stretchability that results in slight to moderate loss of range of motion.

Weakness   Refers to a range of muscle strength from zero to fair.

Planes of Body Motion

2

Planes of the Body

The mid-sagittal (or median) plane is a vertical plane extending in an anteroposterior direction, dividing the body into right and left parts. It is effectively the forward and backward movement plane. A sagittal plane is any plane parallel to the median plane. (Sagitta is Latin for 'arrow'.)

The coronal (or frontal) plane is a vertical plane that divides the body into anterior and posterior portions. It lies at right angles to the sagittal plane and is effectively the side movement plane.

The transverse (or horizontal) plane is a horizontal cross-section, dividing the body into upper and lower sections. It lies at right angles to the other two planes and is effectively the rotational movement plane.

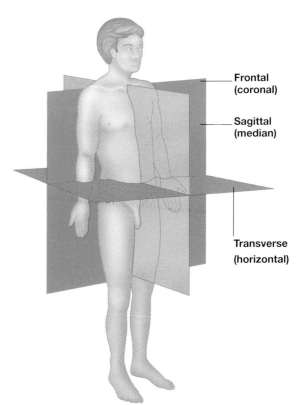

Frontal (coronal)

Sagittal (median)

Transverse (horizontal)

Figure 2.1: Planes of the body.

Terms to Describe Movement

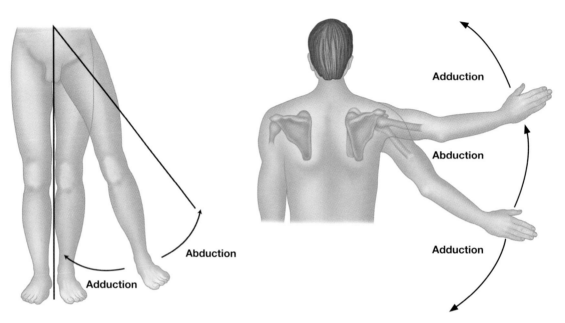

Figure 2.2: Abduction – Movement away from the midline of the body (or a return from adduction).

Figure 2.3: Adduction – Movement towards the midline of the body (or a return from abduction).

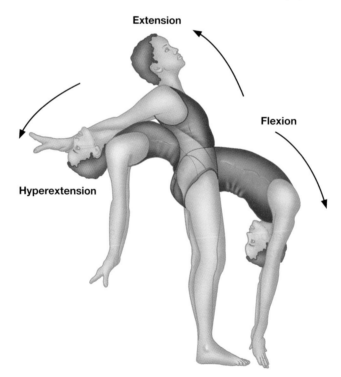

Figure 2.4: Extension – Movement that straightens or increases the angle between the bones or between parts of the body. (Hyperextension is extreme or excessive extension beyond the normal range.) Flexion – Movement that involves bending, e.g. the spine bending forwards.

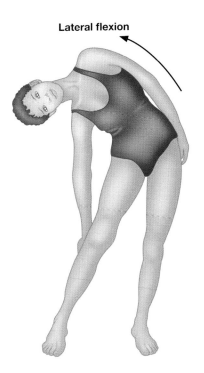

Figure 2.5: Lateral flexion – Bending of the body or head sideways in the coronal plane.

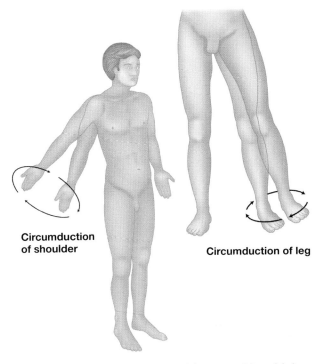

Figure 2.6: Circumduction – Movement in which the distal end of a bone moves in a circle, while the proximal end remains relatively stable. It combines flexion, extension, abduction and adduction.

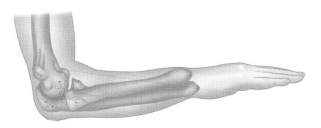

Figure 2.7: Pronation – Medial rotation of the forearm to turn the palm of the hand down to face the floor, or to face posteriorly from the anatomical position.

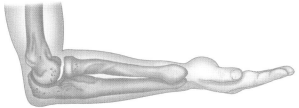

Figure 2.8: Supination – Lateral rotation of the forearm to turn the palm of the hand up to face the ceiling, or to face anteriorly from the anatomical position.

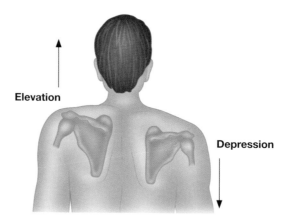

Figure 2.9: Elevation – Movement of a part of the body upwards in the frontal plane.

Figure 2.10: Depression – Movement of an elevated part of the body downwards to its original position.

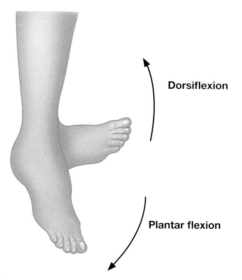

Figure 2.11: Plantar flexion – Pointing the toes downwards.

Figure 2.12: Dorsiflexion – Pointing the toes upwards.

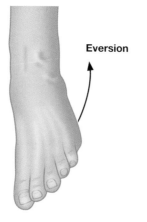

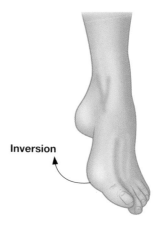

Figure 2.13: Eversion – Turning the sole of the foot outwards. Eversion is part of a movement known as pronation.

Figure 2.14: Inversion – Turning the sole of the foot inwards. Inversion is part of a movement known as supination.

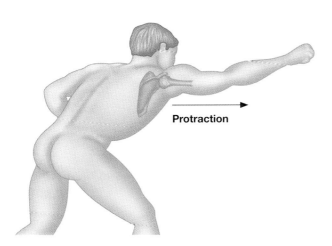

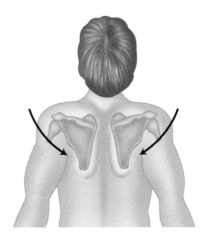

Figure 2.15: Protraction – Drawing out and lengthening of the scapula away from the midline. Movement forwards in the transverse plane.

Figure 2.16: Retraction – Drawing back and shortening of the scapula towards the midline. Movement backwards in the transverse plane.

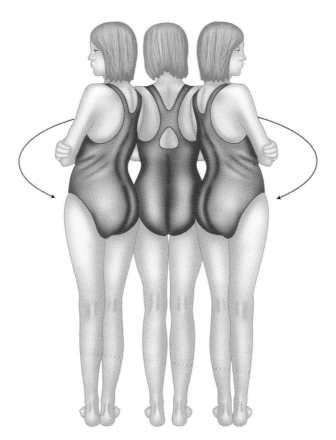

Figure 2.17: Rotation – Turning around a fixed axis. Medial rotation is turning in towards the midline. Lateral rotation is turning out away from the midline.

Muscles and Function

3

The human body contains over 215 pairs of skeletal muscles, which make up approximately 40% of its weight. Skeletal muscles are so named because most attach to and move the skeleton, and so are responsible for movement of the body.

Skeletal muscles have an abundant supply of blood vessels and nerves, which is directly related to contraction, the primary function of skeletal muscle. Each skeletal muscle generally has one main artery to bring nutrients via the blood supply, and several veins to take away metabolic waste (figure 3.1). The blood and nerve supplies generally enter the centre of the muscle, but occasionally towards one end, which eventually penetrates the endomysium around each muscle fibre.

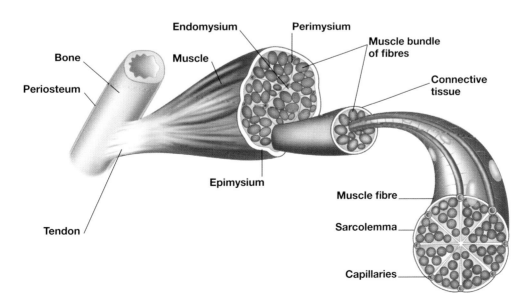

Figure 3.1: A cross-section of skeletal muscle tissue.

Muscle Fibres

The three types of skeletal muscle fibre are: red slow twitch, intermediate fast twitch and white fast twitch. The colour of each is reflected in the amount of myoglobin present, which stores oxygen. The myoglobin is able to increase the rate of oxygen diffusion, so red slow-twitch fibres are able to contract for longer periods, which is particularly useful for endurance events. The white fast-twitch fibres have a lower content of myoglobin. Because these fibres rely on glycogen (energy) reserves, they can contract quickly, but they also fatigue quickly, so are more prevalent in sprinters, or sports in which short, rapid movements are required, such as weightlifting. World-class marathon runners have been reported to possess 93–99% slow-twitch fibres in their gastrocnemius (calf) muscles, whereas world-class sprinters only about 25% in the same muscles (Wilmore and Costill, 1994).

Each skeletal muscle fibre consists of a single cylindrical muscle cell (figure 3.2), which is surrounded by a plasma membrane called the sarcolemma. The sarcolemma features specific openings, which lead to tubes known as transverse (or T) tubules. (The sarcolemma maintains a membrane potential, which allows impulses, specifically to the sarcoplasmic reticulum, to either generate or inhibit contractions.)

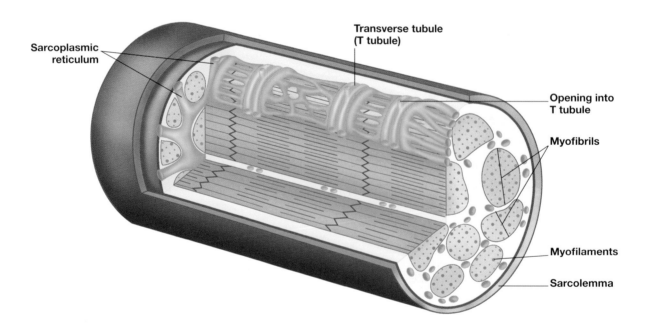

Figure 3.2: Each skeletal muscle fibre is a single cylindrical muscle cell.

An individual skeletal muscle may be made up of hundreds, or even thousands, of muscle fibres bundled together and wrapped in a connective tissue sheath called the epimysium, which gives the muscle its shape, as well as providing a surface against which the surrounding muscles can move. Fascia, connective tissue outside the epimysium, surrounds and separates the muscles. Portions of the epimysium project inwards to divide the muscle into compartments. Each compartment contains a bundle of muscle fibres; each of these bundles is called a fasciculus (from Latin, meaning 'small bundle of twigs') and is surrounded by a layer of connective tissue called the perimysium. Each fasciculus consists of a number of muscle cells, and within the fasciculus, each individual muscle cell is surrounded by the endomysium, a fine sheath of delicate connective tissue.

Types of Muscle

Skeletal muscles come in a variety of shapes (figure 3.3), due to the arrangement of their fasciculus (or 'fascicle' in English), depending on the function of the muscle in relation to its position and action.

- Parallel muscles have their fasciculus running parallel to the long axis of the muscle, e.g. sartorius, biceps brachii.

- Pennate muscles have a short fasciculus, which is attached obliquely to the tendon, and appears feather-shaped, e.g. rectus femoris.

- Convergent (triangular) muscles have a broad origin, with the fasciculus converging towards a single tendon, e.g. pectoralis major.

- Circular (sphincter) muscles have their fasciculus arranged in concentric rings around an opening, e.g. orbicularis oculi.

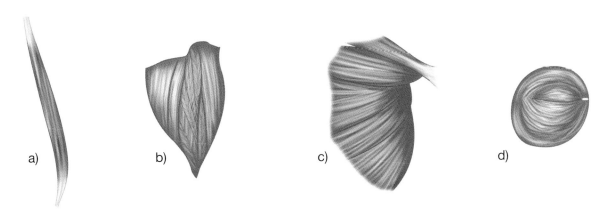

Figure 3.3: Muscle shapes. (a) Parallel; (b) Pennate; (c) Convergent; (d) Circular.

Composition of Muscle Fibres

Each muscle fibre is composed of small structures called muscle fibrils or myofibrils (the Latin prefix myo- means 'muscle'). These myofibrils lie in parallel and give the muscle cell its striated appearance, because they are composed of regularly aligned myofilaments. Myofilaments are chains of protein molecules, which under microscope appear as alternate light and dark bands (figure 3.4). The light isotropic (I) bands are composed of the protein actin. The dark anisotropic (A) bands are composed of the protein myosin. (A third protein called titin has been identified, which accounts for about 11% of the combined muscle protein content.) When a muscle contracts, the actin filaments move between the myosin filaments, forming cross-bridges, which results in the myofibrils shortening and thickening.

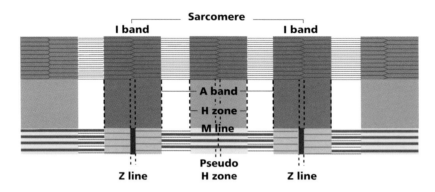

Figure 3.4: The myofilaments within a sarcomere. A sarcomere is bounded at both ends by the Z line, and the M line is the centre of the sarcomere. The I band is composed of actin; the A band of myosin.

Commonly, the epimysium, perimysium and endomysium extend beyond the fleshy part of the muscle – the belly – to form a thick rope-like tendon or broad, flat, sheet-like tendinous tissue, known as an aponeurosis. The tendon and aponeurosis form indirect attachments from muscles to the periosteum of bones or to the connective tissue of other muscles. However, more complex muscles may have multiple attachments, such as the quadriceps (four attachments). So typically a muscle spans a joint and is attached to bones by tendons at both ends. One of the bones remains relatively fixed or stable, while the other end moves as a result of muscle contraction.

Each muscle fibre is innervated (stimulated with nerve impulses) by a single motor nerve fibre, ending near the middle of the muscle fibre. A single motor nerve fibre and all the muscle fibres it supplies is known as a motor unit (figure 3.5). The number of muscle fibres supplied by a single nerve fibre is dependent upon the movement required. When an exact, controlled degree of movement is called upon, such as an eye or finger movement, only a few muscle fibres are supplied; when a grosser movement is required, as when mobilising the large muscles such as the gluteus maximus, several hundred fibres may be recruited.

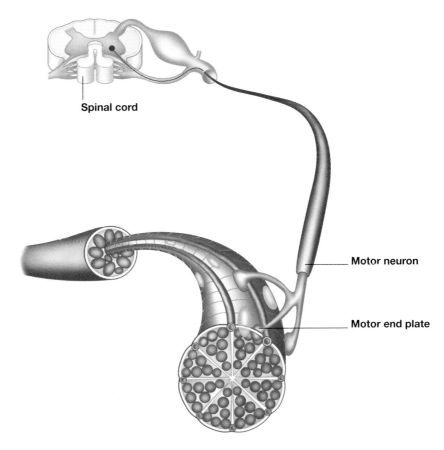

Figure 3.5: A motor unit of a skeletal muscle.

Individual skeletal muscle fibres work on an 'all or nothing' principle, where stimulation of the fibre results in complete contraction of that fibre, or no contraction at all – a fibre cannot be 'slightly contracted'. The overall contraction of any named muscle involves the contraction of a proportion of its fibres at any one time, with other fibres remaining relaxed.

The Physiology of Muscle Contraction

Nerve impulses cause the skeletal muscle fibres at which they terminate, to contract. The junction between a muscle fibre and the motor nerve is known as the neuromuscular junction, and this is where communication between the nerve and the muscle takes place. A nerve impulse arrives at the nerve's endings, called synaptic terminals, close to the sarcolemma. These terminals contain thousands of vesicles filled with a neurotransmitter called acetylcholine (ACh). When a nerve impulse reaches the synaptic terminal, hundreds of these vesicles discharge their ACh. The ACh opens up channels, which allow sodium ions (Na+) to diffuse in. An inactive muscle fibre has a resting potential of about -95 mV. The influx of sodium ions reduces the charge, creating an end plate potential. If the end plate potential reaches the threshold voltage (approximately -50 mV), sodium ions flow in and an action potential is created within the fibre (figure 3.6).

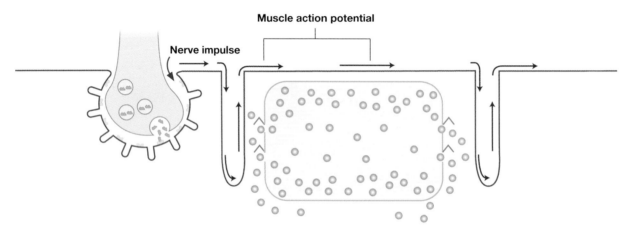

Figure 3.6: Nerve impulse triggering an action potential, resulting in muscle contraction.

No visible change occurs in the muscle fibre during (and immediately following) the action potential. This period, called the latent period, lasts 3–10 milliseconds. Before the latent period is over, the enzyme acetylcholinesterase breaks down the ACh in the neuromuscular junction, the sodium channels close, and the field is cleared for the arrival of another nerve impulse. The resting potential of the fibre is restored by an outflow of potassium ions. The brief period needed to restore the resting potential is called the refractory period.

So how does a muscle fibre shorten? This has been explained best by the sliding filament theory (Huxley and Hanson, 1954), which proposed that muscle fibres receive a nerve impulse (see above) that results in the release of calcium ions stored in the sarcoplasmic reticulum (SR). For muscles to work effectively, energy is required, and this is created by the breakdown of adenosine triphosphate (ATP). This energy allows the calcium ions to bind with the actin and myosin filaments to form a magnetic bond, which causes the fibres to shorten, resulting in a contraction. Muscle action continues until the energy is depleted, at which point calcium is pumped back into the SR, where it is stored until another nerve impulse arrives.

Muscle Reflexes

Skeletal muscles contain specialised sensory units that are sensitive to muscle lengthening (stretching). These sensory units are called muscle spindles and Golgi tendon organs (figure 3.7) and they are important in detecting, responding to and modulating changes in the length of muscle.

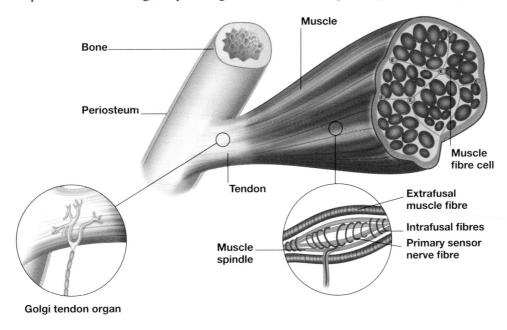

Figure 3.7: Anatomy of a muscle spindle and Golgi tendon organ.

Muscle spindles are made up of spiral threads, called intrafusal muscle fibres, and nerve endings, both encased within a connective tissue sheath, and they monitor the speed at which a muscle is lengthening. If a muscle is lengthening at speed, signals from the intrafusal fibres will fire information via the spinal cord to the nervous system so that a nerve impulse is sent back, causing the lengthening muscle to contract. The signals continuously transfer information to/ from the muscle about position and power (proprioception).

Furthermore, when a muscle is lengthened and held, it will maintain a contractile response as long as the muscle remains stretched. This facility is known as the stretch reflex arc. Muscle spindles will remain stimulated as long as the stretch is held.

The classic clinical example of the stretch reflex is the knee jerk test, which involves activation of the stretch receptors in the patellar tendon, causing reflex contraction of the muscle attached, i.e. the quadriceps.

Whereas the muscle spindles monitor the length of a muscle, the Golgi tendon organs (GTOs) in the muscle tendon can respond to the contraction of a single muscle fibre, since they are so sensitive to tension in the muscle-tendon complex. The GTOs are inhibitory in nature, performing a protective function by reducing the risk of injury. When stimulated, the GTOs inhibit the contracting (agonist) muscles and excite the antagonist muscles. Muscle spindles and GTOs will be discussed in more detail in Chapter 4.

Musculoskeletal Mechanics

Most coordinated movement involves one attachment of a skeletal muscle remaining relatively stationary, while the attachment at the other end moves. The proximal, more fixed, attachment is known as the origin, while the attachment that lies more distally, and moves, is known as the insertion. (However, attachment is now the preferred term for origin and insertion, as it acknowledges that muscles often work so that either end can be fixed while the other end moves.)

Most movements require the application of muscle force, which often is accomplished by agonists (or prime movers), which are primarily responsible for movement and provide most of the force required; antagonists, which have to lengthen to allow for the movement produced by the prime movers, and play a protective role; and synergists, which assist prime movers, and are sometimes involved in fine-tuning the direction of movement. A simple example is the flexion of the elbow (figure 3.8), which requires shortening of the brachialis and biceps brachii (prime movers) and the relaxation of the triceps brachii (antagonist). The brachioradialis acts as the synergist by assisting the brachialis and biceps brachii.

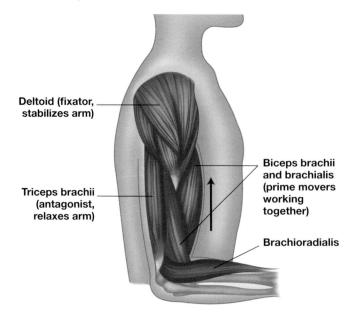

Deltoid (fixator, stabilizes arm)

Triceps brachii (antagonist, relaxes arm)

Biceps brachii and brachialis (prime movers working together)

Brachioradialis

Figure 3.8: Flexion of the elbow. The brachialis and biceps brachii act as the prime movers, the triceps brachii as the antagonist, and the brachioradialis as the synergist.

Skeletal muscles can be broadly grouped according to the predominant fibres they contain: Type I or Type II.

- Type I fibres (slow twitch). These appear red due to the presence of the oxygen-binding protein myoglobin. Muscles which behave tonically (posturally) have a larger number of slow twitch, or Type I fibres. They are fatigue resistant and work at low loads, so are suited to supporting the body against gravity.

- Type II fibres (fast twitch). These are mainly white due to the absence of myoglobin and a reliance on glycolytic enzymes. Muscles with greater proportions of fast twitch, or Type II fibres, are considered to be phasic. However, Type II fibres can be further classified into Type IIa, which are less fatigueable and have aerobic properties, and Type IIb, which are more fatigueable and have anaerobic properties.

As research progresses, it is becoming clearer that muscles do not always behave in such clearly defined ways. Indeed, muscles that have been thought of as operating exclusively tonically have been found to modulate their activity phasically under certain conditions.

Muscle movement can be broken down into three types of contraction: concentric, eccentric and static (isometric). In many activities – such as running, Pilates and yoga – all three types of contraction may occur to produce smooth, coordinated movement.

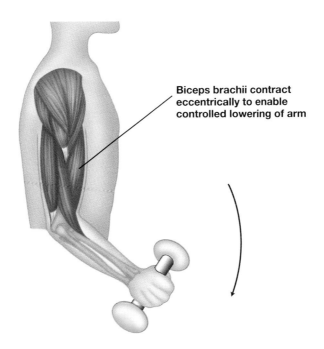

Biceps brachii contract eccentrically to enable controlled lowering of arm

Figure 3.9: An example of eccentric contraction is the action of the biceps brachii when the elbow is extended to lower a heavy weight. Here, biceps brachii is controlling the movement by gradually lengthening in order to resist gravity.

A muscle's principal action – shortening, where the muscle attachments move closer together – is referred to as a concentric contraction (see figure 3.9). Because joint movement is produced, concentric contractions are also considered dynamic contractions. An example is lifting an object, whereby the biceps brachii contracts concentrically, the elbow joint flexes and the hand moves up towards the shoulder.

A movement is considered to be an eccentric contraction where the muscle may exert a force while lengthening. As with a concentric contraction, because joint movement is produced, this is also referred to as a dynamic contraction. The actin filaments are pulled further from the centre of the sarcomere, effectively stretching it. An example of an eccentric contraction is the action of the biceps brachii when the elbow is extended to lower a heavy weight. Here, biceps brachii is controlling the movement by gradually lengthening in order to resist gravity.

When a muscle acts without moving, a force is generated but the length of the muscle remains unchanged. This is known as a static (isometric) contraction. An example of a static contraction is holding a heavy weight, with the elbow stationary and bent at 90 degrees.

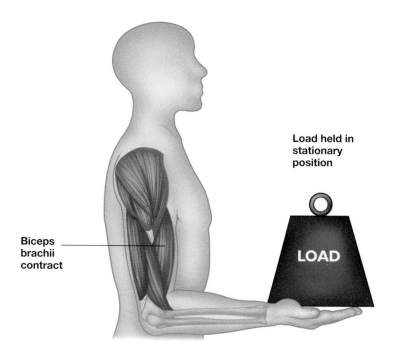

Figure 3.10: An example of static (isometric) contraction, where a heavy weight is held, with the elbow stationary and bent at 90 degrees.

Theory of Muscle Energy Techniques

4

Physical therapists have a toolbox of various techniques that they can employ to help release and relax muscles, which will then assist the patient's body to promote the healing mechanisms. A muscle energy technique is one of those tools that if used correctly can have a major influence on the patient's wellbeing.

Muscle energy techniques (METs) are a form of osteopathic manipulative diagnosis and treatment in which the patient's muscles are actively used on request, from a precisely controlled position, in a specific direction, and against a distinctly executed counterforce. These techniques were first described in 1948 by Fred Mitchell, Sr, DO.

METs are unique in their application, as the patient is providing the initial effort and the practitioner is just facilitating the process. The primary force is from the contraction of the patient's soft tissues (muscles), which is then utilised to assist and correct the presenting musculoskeletal dysfunction.

Muscle energy techniques are generally classified as a direct form of technique as opposed to indirect, since the use of muscular effort is from a controlled position, in a specific direction, against a distant counterforce that is usually offered by the practitioner.

Benefits of METs

The concept I try to teach my students about METs is that one of their benefits is that they are used to normalise joint range, rather than to improve one's flexibility. This might sound counter-intuitive; what I am saying is if, for example, your patient cannot rotate their neck (cervical spine) to the right as far as they can to the left, they have a restriction of the cervical spine in a right rotation. The normal range of rotation for the cervical spine is 80 degrees, but let's say they can rotate to the right only 70 degrees. This is where METs come in. After the MET technique has been employed on the tight restrictive muscles, hopefully the cervical spine will then be capable of rotating to 80 degrees – the patient has made all the effort and you, the practitioner, have encouraged the cervical spine into further right rotation. You have now improved the joint range to 'normal'. This is not stretching in the strictest sense – even though the overall flexibility has been improved, it is only to the point of achieving what is considered to be a normal joint range.

Depending on the context and the variation of MET employed, the objectives of METs can include:

- Restoring normal tone in hypertonic muscles
- Strengthening weak muscles
- Preparing muscles for subsequent stretching
- Increasing joint mobility
- Boosting local circulation
- Improving musculoskeletal function

Restoring Normal Tone in Hypertonic Muscles

Through the simple process of METs, we as physical therapists try to achieve a relaxation in the hypertonic shortened muscles. If we think of a joint as being limited in its range of motion (ROM), then through the initial identification of the hypertonic structures, we can employ the techniques demonstrated in this book to help achieve normality in the tissues. Certain types of massage therapy can also help us achieve this relaxation effect, and generally an MET is applied in conjunction with massage therapy. I personally feel that massage with motion is one of the best tools a physical therapist has.

Strengthening Weak Muscles

METs can be used in the strengthening of weak or even flaccid muscles, as the patients are asked to contract the muscles prior to the lengthening process. The therapist should be able to modify the MET by asking the patient to contract the muscle that has been classified as weak, against a resistance applied by the therapist (isometric contraction), the timing of which can be varied. For example, the patient can be asked to resist the movement using approximately 20–30% of their maximum capability for 5 to 10–15 seconds. They are then asked to repeat the process 5–8 times, resting for 10–15 seconds between repetitions. The patient's performance can be noted and improved over time.

Preparing Muscles for Subsequent Stretching

In certain circumstances, what sport your patient participates in will be determined by what range of motion they have at their joints. Everybody can improve their flexibility, and METs can be used to help achieve this goal. Remember that the focus of METs is to try to improve the 'normal' range of motion of a joint.

If you want to improve the patient's flexibility past the point of 'normal', a more aggressive MET approach might be recommended. This could be in the form of asking the patient to contract a bit firmer than the standard 10–20% of the muscle's capability. For example, we can ask the patient to contract using, say, 40–70% of the muscle's capability. This increased contraction will help stimulate more motor units to fire, causing an increased stimulation of the GTO. This will then have the effect of relaxing more of the muscle, allowing it to be lengthened even further. Either way, once an MET has been incorporated into the treatment plan, a flexibility programme can follow.

Increasing Joint Mobility

One of my favourite sayings when I teach muscle testing courses is: 'A stiff joint can become a tight muscle and a tight muscle can become a stiff joint.' Does this not make perfect sense?

When you use an MET correctly, it is one of the best ways to improve the mobility of the joint, even though you are relaxing the muscles initially. The focus of the MET is to get the patient to contract the muscles; this subsequently causes a relaxation period, allowing a greater range of motion to be achieved within that specific joint.

Boosting Local Circulation

It must go without saying that if you have applied some soft tissue techniques to a dysfunctional area, there has to be an improvement in circulation. As you get the patient to contract for 10 seconds and relax, then repeat the process a few times, this approach will automatically encourage blood flow into that area.

Improving Musculoskeletal Function

As you make your way through each chapter, you will notice a chart which you can use to identify specific areas that need an MET treatment. In the first instance, you are shown how to assess and use METs to treat dysfunctions of the soft tissues in the upper body. Once you have assessed and treated the upper body, the same approach can be applied to the lower body and the trunk musculature. This approach, if utilised on a regular basis, will have a major effect on a person's whole musculoskeletal function.

Physiological Effects of METs

'Postural deviations' are described in Chapters 5 and 6. By using the techniques demonstrated in this book, we will initially identify which muscles are classified as 'short' and what effects this has on one's body position. Once these muscles have been identified, either through observation or the tests described in this book, we will then be able to use an MET to help correct these dysfunctions, and a corrective treatment plan can be designed.

There are two main effects of METs and these are explained by virtue of two distinct physiological processes:

- Post-isometric relaxation (PIR)
- Reciprocal inhibition (RI)

When we use MET, certain neurological influences occur. Before we discuss the main process of PIR/RI, we need to consider the two types of receptor involved in the stretch reflex:

- Muscle spindles, which are sensitive to change in length and speed of change in muscle fibres.
- Golgi tendon organs (GTOs), which detect prolonged change in tension.

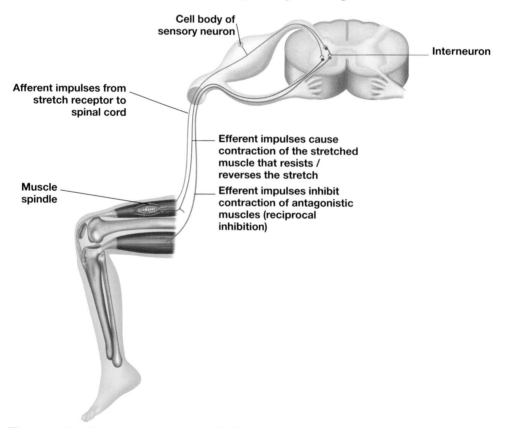

Figure 4.1: The stretch reflex arc and reciprocal inhibition (RI).

Stretching the muscle causes an increase in the impulses transmitted from the muscle spindle to the posterior horn cell (PHC) of the spinal cord. In turn, the anterior horn cell (AHC) transmits an increase in motor impulses to the muscle fibres, creating a protective tension to resist the stretch. However, increased tension after a few seconds is sensed within the GTOs, which transmit impulses to the PHC. These impulses have an inhibitory effect on the increased motor stimulus at the AHC.

This inhibitory effect causes a reduction in motor impulses and consequent relaxation. This implies that the prolonged stretch of the muscles will increase the stretching capability because of the protective relaxation of the GTOs overriding the protective contraction due to the muscle spindles. However, a fast stretch of the muscle spindles will cause immediate muscle contraction and since it is not sustained there will be no inhibitory action. This is known as the basic reflex arc.

PIR results from a neurological feedback through the spinal cord to the muscle itself when an isometric contraction is sustained, causing a reduction in tone of the muscle, which has been contracted. This reduction in tone lasts for approximately 20 to 25 seconds, during which time the tissues can be more easily moved to a new resting length.

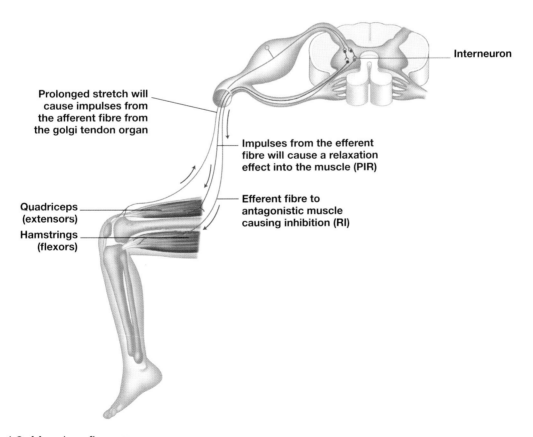

Interneuron

Prolonged stretch will cause impulses from the afferent fibre from the golgi tendon organ

Impulses from the efferent fibre will cause a relaxation effect into the muscle (PIR)

Quadriceps (extensors)

Efferent fibre to antagonistic muscle causing inhibition (RI)

Hamstrings (flexors)

Figure 4.2: Muscle reflex arc.

When RI is employed, the reduction in tone relies on the physiological inhibiting effect of antagonists on the contraction of a muscle. When the motor neurons of the contracting agonist muscle receive excitatory impulses from the afferent pathway, the motor neurons of the opposing antagonist muscle receive inhibitory impulses at the same time, which prevent it contracting. It follows that contraction or extended stretch of the agonist muscle must elicit relaxation or inhibit the antagonist; also, a fast stretch of the agonist will facilitate a contraction of the agonist.

The refractory period of about 20 seconds occurs with RI; however, RI is thought to be less powerful than PIR. Therapists need to be able to use both approaches, because at times use of the agonist may be inappropriate due to pain or injury. Since with an MET the amount of force used is minimal, the risk of injury or tissue damage will be reduced.

METs can be used for both acute and chronic conditions. Acute involves anything that is obviously acute in terms of symptoms, pain or spasm, as well as anything that has emerged during the previous three to four weeks. Anything older and of a less obviously acute nature is regarded as chronic in determining which variation of MET is suitable.

MET Method of Application

- The patient's limb is taken to the point where resistance is felt; this is known as the restriction barrier or the point of bind. It can be more comfortable for the patient if you bring back the area that you are going to treat to a point slightly short of the point of bind, especially if tissues are in a chronic state.
- The patient is asked to isometrically contract the muscle to be treated (PIR) or the antagonist (RI), using approximately 10–20% of the muscle's strength capability against a resistance that is applied by the therapist.
- The patient should be using the agonist if the method of approach is PIR; this will release the tight shortened structures directly.
- If the RI method of MET is used, the patient is asked to contract the antagonist isometrically; this will induce a relaxation effect in the opposite muscle group (agonist) that would still be classified as the tight and shortened structures. See the PIR example below.
- The patient is asked to slowly introduce an isometric contraction, lasting between 10 and 12 seconds, avoiding any jerking of the treated area. This contraction as explained is the time necessary to load the GTOs, which allows them to become active and to influence the intrafusal fibres from the muscle spindles. This has the effect of overriding the influence from the muscle spindles, which inhibits muscle tone. The therapist has then the opportunity to take the affected area to a new position with minimal effort.
- The contraction by the patient should cause no discomfort or strain.
- The patient is told to relax fully by taking a deep breath in, and as they breathe out, the

therapist passively takes the specific joint that lengthens the hypertonic muscle to a new position, which therefore normalises joint range.

■ After an isometric contraction, which induces a PIR, there is a relaxation period of 15–30 seconds; this period can be the perfect time to stretch the tissues to their new resting length.

■ Repeat this process until no further progress is made (normally 3–4 times) and hold the final resting position for approximately 25–30 seconds. It is considered that the 25–30 seconds period is enough time for the neurological system to lock onto this new resting position.

■ This type of technique is excellent for relaxing and releasing tone in tight, shortened soft tissues.

'Point of Bind' or the 'Restriction Barrier'

Throughout this book the word 'bind' will be mentioned numerous times. The restriction barrier is the first place in which bind is felt by the palpating hand/fingers of the therapist.

Through experience and continual practising, the therapist will be able to palpate a resistance of the soft tissues as the affected area is gently taken into the position in which a bind is felt. This position of bind is not the position of stretch – it is the position just before the point of stretch. The therapist should be able to feel the difference and not wait for the patient to say when they feel a stretch has occurred.

In most applications of METs, the position of bind or just short of the position of bind is the preferred method in which an MET is utilised.

Clearly, an MET is quite a mild form of stretching when compared to other techniques, so one can assume it is therefore more appropriate to the rehabilitation process. It should be borne in mind that most problems with muscle shortening will occur in postural muscles. Since these muscles are composed predominantly of slow-twitch fibres, a milder form of stretching is perhaps more appropriate.

Acute and Chronic

The soft tissues that you treat using METs are generally classified as either acute or chronic, and this tends to relate to tissues that have had some form of strain or trauma. If you feel the presenting condition is relatively acute (occurring within the last three weeks), the isometric contraction can be performed at the point of bind. After the patient has contracted the muscle isometrically for the duration of 10 seconds, the therapist then takes the affected area to the new point of bind.

In chronic conditions (persisting for more than three weeks), the isometric contraction starts from a position just before the point of bind. After the patient has contracted the muscle for 10 seconds, the therapist then goes through the point of bind and encourages the specific area into the new position.

PIR versus RI

How much pain the patient is presenting with is generally the deciding factor in determining which method to initially apply. The PIR method is usually the technique of choice for muscles that are classified as 'short' and 'tight', as it is these muscles that are initially contracted in the process of releasing and relaxing.

However, on occasion the patient experiences discomfort when the agonist, i.e. the shortened structure, is contracted; in this case it would seem more appropriate to contract the opposite muscle group (antagonist), as this would reduce the patient's perception of pain, but still induce a relaxation in the painful tissues. Hence, the use of the RI method, using the antagonists, which are usually pain free, will generally be the first choice if there is increased sensitivity in the primary shortened tissues.

When the patient's initial pain has been reduced by the appropriate treatment, PIR techniques can be incorporated (as explained earlier, PIR uses an isometric contraction of the tight shortened structures, as compared to the antagonists being used in the RI method). To some extent, the main factor in deciding the best approach is whether the sensitive tissue is in the acute stage or chronic stage.

In my experience of using PIR and RI on a regular basis, I have found that the best results of lengthening the hypertonic structures are achieved with PIR (patient has no pain during this technique). However, once I have performed the PIR method, if I feel more range of motion is needed in the shortened tight tissue, I bring into play the antagonists using the RI method for approximately two more repetitions. This approach for my patients has had the desired effect of improving the overall range of motion.

PIR Example

The following is an example of a PIR method of MET treatment. Place your left (or right) hand onto a blank piece of paper and, with the hand open as much as possible, draw around the fingers and the thumb. (Remember doing this as a child?)

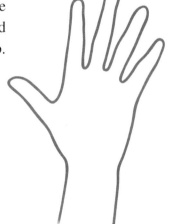

Figure 4.3: PIR method of MET treatment for the adductor pollicis muscle.

We are now going to employ a PIR method of MET treatment for the adductor pollicis muscle. (Pollicis relates to the thumb, or pollex). Actively abduct the thumb as far as you can so a sense of bind is achieved. Next, place the fingers of your right hand on top of the left thumb and, using an isometric contraction, adduct your thumb against the downward pressure of the fingers, so that an isometric contraction is achieved. Apply this pressure for 10 seconds. Once the time has passed, breath in and on the exhalation, passively take the thumb into further abduction (do not force the thumb).

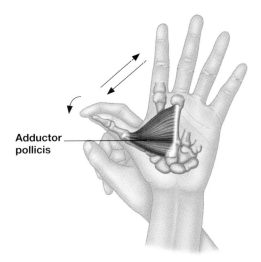

Adductor pollicis

Figure 4.4: Adducting the thumb against a resistance applied by the opposite hand.

Repeat this sequence two more times and on the last repetition, hold the isometric contraction for at least 20–25 seconds. Place your hand back on the piece of paper and draw around it again; hopefully you will see that the thumb abducts further than before.

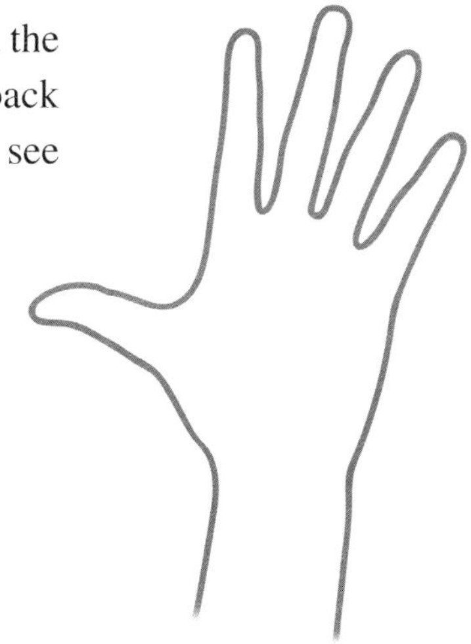

Figure 4.5: The hand redrawn after the MET treatment using PIR.

Understanding the Meaning of the Word 'Tight'

It can be very confusing for therapists to understand the meaning of the word 'tight', as it is interchangeable with the term 'short', or it may be used as an alternative to the term 'taut'. For example, an inexperienced therapist might palpate tissue and automatically say that the tissue feels tight to them; what they might not understand when they are palpating the tissue is whether the tissue has shortened and feels tight, or the tissue is on stretch and subsequently feels tight.

Let's look at this another way – I will use an example in a clinic setting. When we treat the upper trapezius, we might say that the muscle palpates as tight, due to the fact this is a postural muscle, which has a tendency to shorten and subsequently palpate as tight. When we come on to the lower fibres of the trapezius, again we might be tempted to use the word 'tight', as these fibres could feel similar to the tissues of the upper trapezius. However, what you might be palpating, in fact, is the taut tissue of the lower trapezius, due to it being in a stretched position and subsequently held in a weakened position.

In reality, if you treat the upper and lower trapezius using the same techniques, one component of the muscle might improve, whereas the other might remain the same, or even deteriorate further.

Remember that lengthening the tight shortened structure (antagonist) initially can assist in shortening the already stretched and lengthened tissue, which can have the effect of resolving the muscle imbalance.

As Kendall (2010) points out: 'Weakness permits a position of deformity, but shortness creates a position of deformity.' In other words,

> *'A tight muscle will pull the joint into a dysfunctional position*
> *and the weak muscle will allow it to happen.'*

Muscle Imbalances

Posture can be defined as the attitude or position of the body (Thomas, 1997) and according to Martin (2002) should fulfil three functions:

- It must maintain the alignment of the body's segments in any position: supine, prone, sitting, quadruped and standing.
- It must anticipate change to allow engagement in voluntary, goal-directed movements, such as reaching and stepping.
- It must react to unexpected perturbations or disturbances in balance.

From the above, it can be seen that posture is an active as well as a purely static state and that it is synonymous with balance. Optimal posture must be maintained at all times, not only when holding static positions (e.g. sitting, standing) but also during movement.

If optimal posture and postural control is to be encouraged during exercise performance, the principles of good static posture must be fully appreciated. Once this is understood, poor posture can be identified and corrective strategies adopted.

- Good posture is the state of muscular and skeletal balance that protects the supporting structures of the body against injury or progressive deformity, irrespective of the attitude (e.g. erect, lying, squatting, stooping) in which these structures are working or resting.

- Poor posture is a faulty relationship of the various parts of the body, which produces increased strain on the supporting structures and in which there is less efficient balance of the body over its base of support.

The neuromuscular system as we know is made up of slow-twitch and fast-twitch muscle fibres, each having a different role in the body's function. Fast-twitch fibres are for powerful, gross movements, whereas slow-twitch fibres are for sustained low-level activity, such as maintaining correct posture. Muscles can also be broken down into two further categories – postural and phasic.

Postural and Phasic Muscles

Previous authors have suggested that muscles that have a stabilising function (postural) have a tendency to shorten when stressed, and other muscles that play a more active/moving role (phasic) have a tendency to lengthen and become inhibited. The muscles that tend to shorten have a primary postural role, and we can use this book to identify the shortened tight structures. There are some exceptions to the rule that certain muscles follow the pattern of becoming shortened while others become lengthened – some muscles are capable of modifying their structure.

For example, certain authors suggest that the scalenes are postural in nature and some suggest that they are phasic. We know that, depending on what dysfunction is present within the muscle framework, on specific testing one can find the scalenes to be held in a shortened position and tight, but sometimes when they are tested they can be found to be lengthened and weakened.

There is a distinction between postural and phasic muscles; however, many muscles can display characteristics of both and contain a mixture of Type I and Type II fibres. The hamstring muscles, for example, have a postural stabilising function, yet are polyarticular (cross more than one joint) and are notoriously prone to shortening.

	Postural	**Phasic**
Function	Posture	Movement
Muscle type	Type I	Type II
Fatigue	Late	Early
Reaction	Shortening	Lengthening

Table 5.1: Lengthening and shortening of muscles.

Postural Muscles
Also known as tonic muscles, these muscles have an antigravity role and are therefore heavily involved in the maintenance of posture. Slow-twitch fibres are more suited to maintaining posture; they are capable of sustained contraction and generally become shortened and subsequently tight.

Postural muscles are slow-twitch dominant, due to their resistance to fatigue, and are innervated by a smaller motor neuron. They therefore have a lower excitability threshold, which means the nerve impulse will reach the postural muscle before the phasic muscle. With this sequence of innervation, the postural muscle will inhibit the phasic (antagonist) muscle, thus reducing its contractile potential and activation.

When your muscles are placed under faulty or repetitive loading, the postural muscles will shorten and the phasic muscles will weaken. This consequently alters their length-tension relationship, which will directly affect posture, as the surrounding muscles displace the soft tissues and the skeletal system.

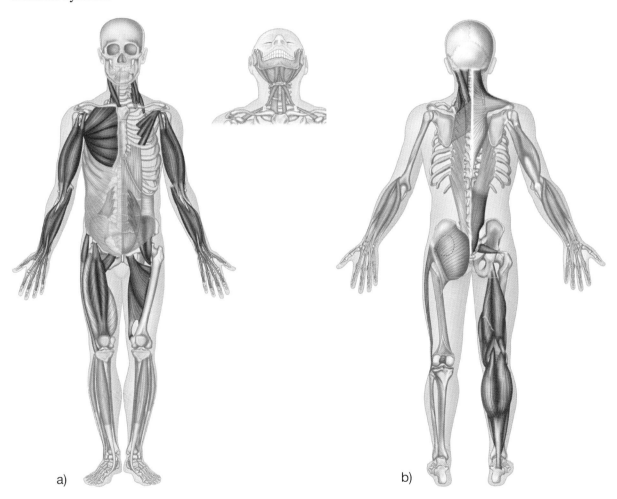

a)   b)

Figure 5.1: Postural-phasic muscles, a) anterior view, b) posterior view. Purple muscles predominantly postural, and green muscles predominantly phasic.

Phasic Muscles

Movement is the main function of phasic muscles. These muscles are often relatively more superficial than postural muscles and tend to span several joints (polyarticular). They are composed of predominantly fast-twitch Type II fibres and are under voluntary reflex control.

A tight muscle often results in inhibition of the phasic muscle, whose function becomes weakened as a result. The relationship between a tightness-prone muscle and its weakness-prone muscle is one way. As the tightness-prone muscle becomes tighter and subsequently stronger, this causes an inhibition of the weakness-prone muscle, resulting in its lengthening and consequent weakening. The division of the muscles into predominantly postural and predominantly phasic is shown in table 5.2.

Predominantly postural muscles	Predominantly phasic muscles
Shoulder girdle	
Pectoralis major/minor	Rhomboids
Levator scapulae	Lower trapezius
Upper trapezius	Mid trapezius
Biceps brachii	Seratus anterior
Neck extensors: Scalenes / Cervical erectors / Sternocleido-mastoid	Triceps brachii
	Neck flexors: Supra- and infrahyoid / Longus colli
Lower arm	
Wrist flexors	Wrist extensors
Trunk	
Lumbar and cervical erectors	Thoracic erectors
Quadratus lumborum	Abdominals
Pelvis	
Biceps femoris / Semitendinosus / Semimembranosus	Vastus medialis
Iliopsoas	Vastus lateralis
ITB	Gluteus maximus
Rectus femoris	Gluteus minimus and medius
Adductors	
Piriformis / Tensor fasciae latae	
Lower leg	
Gastrocnemius / Soleus	Tibialis anterior / Peroneals

Table 5.2: Phasic and postural muscles of the body.

Muscle Activity Before and After Stretching

Let's look at some EMG studies of trunk muscle activity before and after stretching hypertonic muscles, in this case the erector spinae.

In table 5.3 the hypertonic erector spinae are indicated as being active during trunk flexion. After stretching, the erector spinae are suppressed both in trunk flexion (which allowed greater activation of the rectus abdominis) and in trunk extension.

Muscle	First recording			Second recording		
Rectus abdominis						
Erector spinae						

Table 5.3: EMG recordings of muscle activity. Reproduced from Hammer, W. I. 'Functional Soft Tissue Examination and Treatment by Manual Methods.' Permission sought.

Effects of Muscle Imbalance

The research results of Janda (1983) indicate that tight or overactive muscles not only hinder the agonist through Sherrington's law of reciprocal inhibition, but also become active in movements that they are not normally associated with.

Note: This is the reason, when trying to correct a musculoskeletal imbalance, you would encourage lengthening of an overactive muscle using an MET, prior to attempting to strengthen a weak elongated muscle.

If these muscle imbalances are not addressed, the body will be forced into a compensatory position, which increases the stress placed on the musculoskeletal system, eventually leading to tissue breakdown, irritation and injury. You are now in a vicious circle of musculoskeletal deterioration as the tonic muscles shorten and the phasic muscles lengthen (figure 5.1).

Muscle imbalances are ultimately reflected in posture. As mentioned earlier, postural muscles are innervated by a smaller motor neuron and therefore have a lower excitability threshold. Since the nerve impulse reaches the postural muscle before the phasic muscle, the postural muscle will inhibit the phasic (antagonist) muscle, thus reducing the contractile potential and activation.

When muscles are subject to faulty or repetitive loading, the tonic muscles shorten and the phasic muscles weaken, thus altering their length-tension relationship. Consequently, posture is directly affected because the surrounding muscles displace the soft tissues and the skeleton.

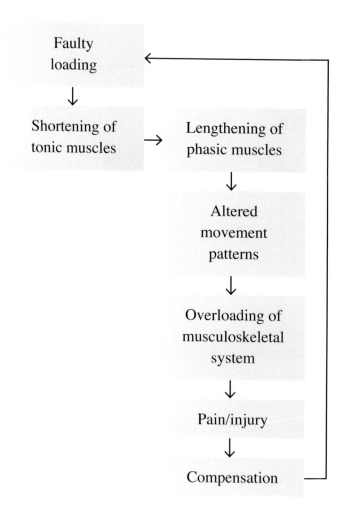

Table 5.4: The vicious circle of musculoskeletal deterioration.

Core Muscle Relationships

As the incidences of lower back pain (LBP) seem to be on the increase, we will need to look at and understand the muscular relationships that affect core and lumbopelvic stability and how METs can be incorporated into the assessment and treatment plan.

The pelvis, or sacroiliac (SI) joint to be more precise, has two main factors that affect its stability:

■ Form closure
■ Force closure

Form Closure

Form closure arises from the anatomical alignment of the bones of the ilium and the sacrum, where the sacrum forms a kind of keystone between the wings of the pelvis.

The sacroiliac joint transfers large loads and its shape is adapted to this task. The articular surfaces are relatively flat and this helps to transfer compression forces and bending movements. However, a relatively flat joint is vulnerable to shear forces. The sacroiliac joint is protected from these forces in three ways. First, the sacrum is wedge-shaped and thus is stabilised by the innominates. Second, in contrast to other synovial joints, the articular cartilage is not smooth but rather irregular. Third, a frontal dissection through the sacroiliac joint reveals cartilage-covered bone extensions protruding into the joint – the so-called ridges and grooves. They seem irregular, but are in fact complementary, and this serves to stabilise the joint when compression is applied.

Force Closure

If the articular surfaces of the sacrum and the innominates fit together with perfect form closure, mobility would be practically impossible. However, form closure of the sacroiliac joint is not perfect and mobility is possible, albeit small, and therefore stabilisation during loading is required. This is achieved by increasing compression across the joint at the moment of loading. The anatomical structures responsible for this are the ligaments, muscles and fasciae. When the sacroiliac joint is compressed, friction of the joint increases and consequently augments form closure. The mechanism of compression of the sacroiliac joints due to extra forces is called force closure.

Sacroiliac stability

Several ligaments, muscles and fascial systems contribute to force closure of the pelvis. When working efficiently, the shear forces between the innominates and the sacrum are adequately controlled and loads can be transferred between the trunk, pelvis and legs.

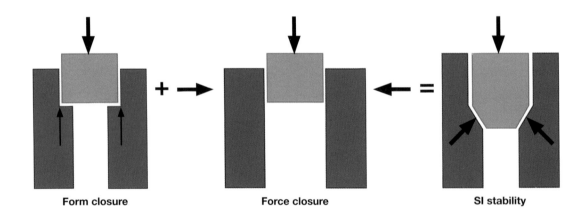

Figure 6.1: The relationship between form and force closure, and SI stability.

In which position is the pelvic girdle the most stable? Studies have shown that sacral nutation occurs when moving from sitting to standing, and that full nutation occurs during forward or backward bending of the trunk. This motion tightens the major ligaments (sacrotuberous, sacrospinous, interosseus) of the posterior pelvis and this tension increases the compressive force across the sacroiliac joint.

Force Closure Ligaments

The main ligamentous structures that influence force closure are the sacrotuberous ligament (which connects the sacrum to the ischium) and the long dorsal sacroiliac ligament (which connects the third and fourth sacral segments to the posterior superior iliac spine (PSIS)).

Ligaments can increase articular compression when they are tensed or lengthened by the movement of the bones to which they attach. Alternatively, they can increase articular compression when they are tensed by contraction of muscles that insert in them. Tension in the sacrotuberous ligament can be increased by posterior rotation of the innominates relative to the sacrum, by nutation of the sacrum relative to the innominates or by contraction of the muscles that attach to it (biceps femoris, piriformis, gluteus maximus, multifidus).

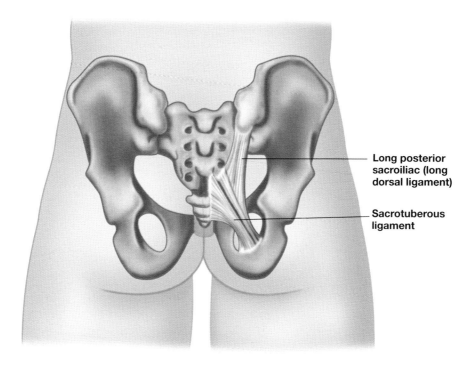

Long posterior sacroiliac (long dorsal ligament)

Sacrotuberous ligament

Figure 6.2: Force closure ligaments.

The main ligamentous restraint to counternutation of the sacrum, or anterior rotation of the innominate, is the long dorsal sacroiliac ligament. This is a relatively less stable position for the pelvis to resist horizontal and/or vertical loading, since the sacroiliac joint is under less compression and is not self-locked.

By themselves, ligaments cannot maintain a stable pelvis – they rely on several muscle systems to assist them. There are two important groups of muscles that contribute to stability of the lower back and pelvis. Collectively they have been called the inner unit (core) and the outer unit (sling systems). The inner unit consists of the transversus abdominis, multifidus, diaphragm and muscles of the pelvic floor – also collectively known as the core, or local stabilisers. The outer unit consists of several slings or systems of muscles (global stabilisers and mobilisers that are anatomically connected and functionally related).

Force Closure Muscles

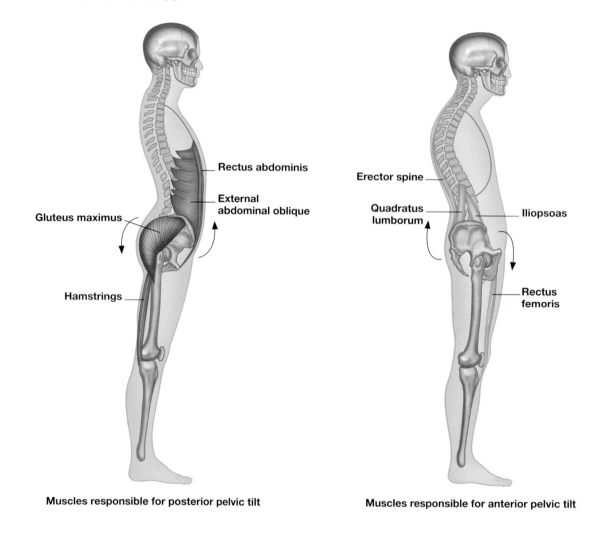

Muscles responsible for posterior pelvic tilt

Muscles responsible for anterior pelvic tilt

Figure 6.3: Anteroposterior pelvic force couples.

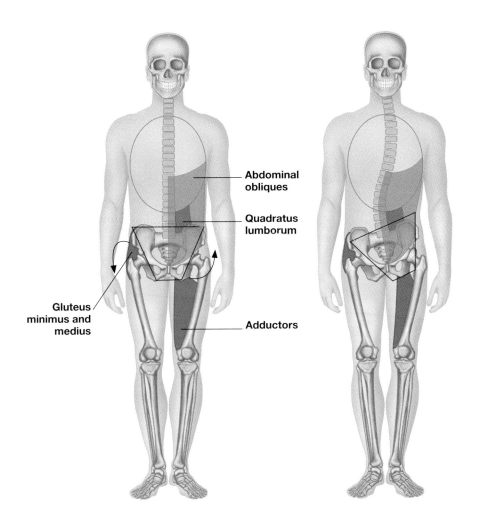

Abdominal obliques

Quadratus lumborum

Gluteus minimus and medius

Adductors

Figure 6.4: Lateral pelvic force couples.

Definition

Force couple – A situation where two forces of equal magnitude, but opposite direction, are applied to an object and pure rotation results (Abernethy et al., 2004).

The Inner Unit: The Core

According to Chek (1999) static stability is 'the ability to remain in one position for a long time without losing good structural alignment'.

Static stability is also often referred to as postural stability, although this might be somewhat misleading since as Martin (2002) states: '… posture is more than just maintaining a position of the body such as standing. Posture is active, whether it is in sustaining an existing posture or moving from one posture to another'.

The core consists of:

- Transversus abdominis (TVA)
- Multifidus
- Diaphragm
- Muscles of the pelvic floor

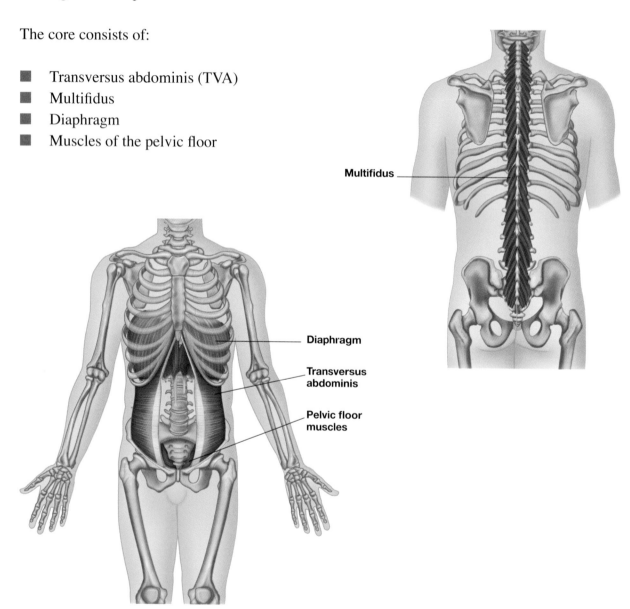

Figure 6.5: The inner unit – the core.

Only the TVA and multifidus will be covered in this book, as these muscles are specifically related to postural and phasic imbalances and are easily palpated by the physical therapist. However, since the diaphragm and muscles of the pelvic floor are difficult to palpate, they will not be discussed.

Transversus Abdominis (TVA)

This is the deepest of the abdominal muscles. It originates at the iliac crest, inguinal ligament, lumbar fascia and the associated cartilage of the inferior six ribs, and attaches to the xiphoid process, linea alba and pubis.

The main action of the TVA is to compress the abdomen via a 'drawing in' of the abdominal wall. This drawing in is observable as a movement of the umbilicus towards the spine. The muscle neither flexes nor extends the spine. Kendall et al. (2010) also state that 'this muscle has no action in lateral flexion except that it acts to … stabilize the linea alba, thereby permitting better action by anterolateral trunk muscles [internal and external obliques]'.

The TVA appears to be the key muscle of the inner unit. Richardson et al. (1999) found that in people without back pain, the TVA fired 30 milliseconds prior to shoulder movements and 110 milliseconds before leg movements. This provides evidence of the key role of the TVA in providing the stability necessary to perform movements of the appendicular skeleton. As the TVA contracts during inspiration it pulls the central tendon inferiorly and flattens, thereby increasing the vertical length of the thoracic cavity and compressing the lumbar multifidus.

Multifidus

The multifidus is the largest and most medial of the lumbar back muscles, and its fibres are centred on each of the lumbar spinous processes. From each spinous process, fibres radiate inferiorly, passing to the transverse processes of the vertebrae two, three, four and five levels below. Those fibres that extend below the level of the last lumbar vertebra (L5) anchor to the ilium and the sacrum.

The importance of the multifidus in producing this extension force is essential to stability of the lumbar spine in acting to resist flexion and shear forces and to control these movements during flexion.

Richardson et al. (1999) identified the lumbar multifidus and the TVA as the key stabilisers of the lumbar spine. Both muscles link in with the thoracolumbar fascia to provide what Richardson et al. referred to as 'a natural, deep muscle corset to protect the back from injury'.

The Outer Unit: The Integrated Sling System

In the past, four systems have been described that comprise the outer unit of muscles – the posterior oblique, the anterior oblique, the longitudinal and the lateral. Although these muscles can be trained individually, effective force closure requires specific co-activation and release for optimal function. The outer unit consists of four systems: Posterior longitudinal; Lateral; Anterior oblique and Posterior oblique.

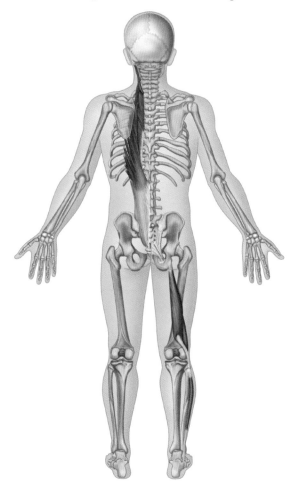

Figure 6.6: Posterior longitudinal system.

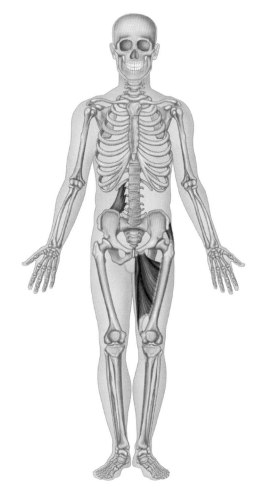

Figure 6.7: Lateral system.

Peroneus longus – the first metatarsal to the head of the fibula

Biceps femoris – the head of the fibula to the ischium

Sacrotuberous ligament – the ischium to the sacrum

Contralateral (opposite) erector spinae – the sacrum to the ilium, costals, vertebrae and cranium

Gluteus medius and minimus (abductors of the hip)

Ipsilateral (same side) adductors of the hip

Contralateral quadratus lumborum

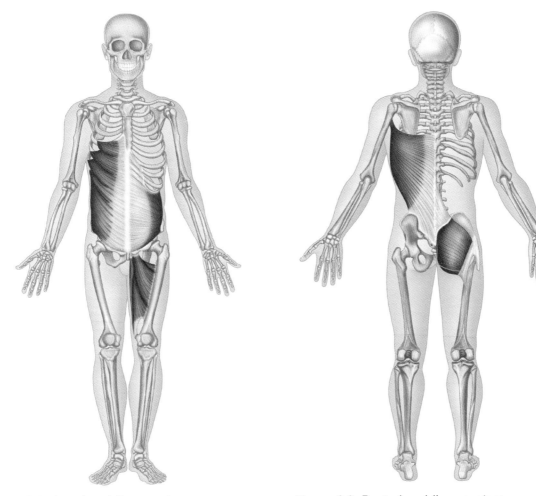

Figure 6.8: Anterior oblique system.   *Figure 6.9: Posterior oblique system.*

Stance leg adductors   Gluteus maximus
Ipsilateral internal obliques   Contralateral latissimus dorsi
Contralateral external obliques   Thoracolumbar fascia

The integrated sling system represents many forces and is composed of several muscles. A muscle may participate in more than one sling, and the slings may overlap and interconnect, depending on the task being demanded. There are several slings of myofascial systems in the outer unit. These include, but are probably not limited to, a coronal sling (having medial and lateral components), a sagittal sling (having anterior and posterior components) and an oblique spiral sling. The hypothesis is that the slings have no beginning or end, but rather connect as necessary to assist in the transference of forces. It is possible that the slings are all part of one interconnected myofascial system, and a sling that is identified during any particular motion could merely be due to the activation of selective parts of the whole sling. (Lee, 2004)

The identification and treatment of a specific muscle dysfunction (such as weakness, inappropriate recruitment, tightness) is important when restoring force closure (second component of stability) and for understanding why parts of a sling may be restricted in motion or lacking in support. Note the following points:

- The four systems of the outer unit are dependent upon the inner unit for the joint stiffness and stability necessary to create an effective force generation platform.

- Failure of the inner unit to work in the presence of outer unit demand often results in muscle imbalance, joint injury and poor performance.

- The outer unit cannot be effectively conditioned by using modern bodybuilding machines, as the specific training using the machines generally does not relate to day-to-day functional movements.

- Effective conditioning of the outer unit should include exercises that require integrated function of the inner and outer units, using movement patterns common to any given client's work or sport environment (Chek, 1999).

Poor Posture

Poor posture may be a result of many varying factors. It may be due to trauma suffered by the body, some form of deformity within the musculoskeletal system, or even faulty loading.

Because sitting has become a position that our bodies maintain for long periods of time (possibly 8+ hours), a majority of today's society are losing the fight against gravity and altering their centre of gravity (COG). With correct posture, the postural muscles are fairly inactive and energy efficient, only responding to disruptions in the balance to maintain an upright position. Therefore, as one moves away from ideal alignment, postural muscle tone is increased, thus increasing energy expenditure.

Sagittal Postural Deviations

Postural deviations can be observed from the sagittal plane, as seen in the following pictures. The text highlights which particular muscles are prone to shortening and becoming tight, and those that are prone to lengthening and becoming weak.

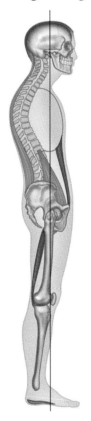

Head:	Forward
Cervical:	Slightly extended
Thoracic:	Lower part straight / upper part flexed
Lumbar:	Flexed (straight)
Pelvis:	Posterior tilt
Hip:	Extended
Knee:	Extended (or flexed)
Ankle:	Slight plantar flexion
Weak and elongated:	Iliopsoas Back extensors (may not be weak)
Short and strong:	Hamstrings

Figure 6.10: Flat-back posture.

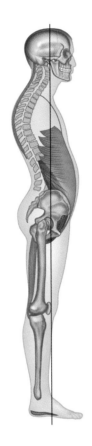

Head:	Forward
Cervical:	Hyperextended
Scapulae:	Abducted
Thoracic:	Hyperkyphosis
Lumbar:	Hyperlordosis
Pelvis:	Anterior tilt
Hip:	Flexed
Knee:	Slightly hyperextended
Ankle:	Slight plantar flexion
Weak and elongated:	Neck flexors
	Upper back
	Hamstrings (may not be weak)
	Obliques
Short and strong:	Neck extensors
	Hip flexors

Figure 6.11: Kyphotic/lordotic posture.

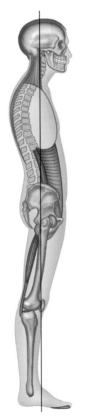

Head:	Forward
Cervical:	Slightly extended
Thoracic:	Flexion (kyphosis)
Lumbar:	Flattened (flexion)
Pelvis:	Posterior tilt
Hip:	Hyperextended and forward
Knee:	Hyperextended
Ankle:	Neutral (pelvis deviation)
Weak and elongated:	Iliopsoas
	Obliques
	Upper back extensors
	Neck flexors
Short and strong:	Hamstrings
	Lower back (not short)
	Upper abdominals

Figure 6.12: Sway-back posture.

Pain Spasm Cycle

Ischaemia will be a primary source of pain in the initial stages of poor posture. The blood flow through a muscle is inversely proportional to the level of contraction or activity, reaching almost zero at 50-60% of contraction. Some studies have indicated that the body could not maintain homeostasis with contractions over 10%.

The weight of the head is approximately 7% of the total body weight (shoulders and arms are around 14%). This means that for an 80 kg man, the head will weigh around 5 to 6 kg. If the head and shoulders move forwards, out of ideal alignment, the activation of the neck extensors is increased dramatically, resulting in restricted blood flow. This prolonged isometric contraction will force the muscles into anaerobic metabolism and increase lactic acid and other irritating metabolite accumulation. If adequate rest is not given, this may initiate a reflex contraction of the already ischaemic muscles. You have now entered the pain spasm cycle (figure 6.13).

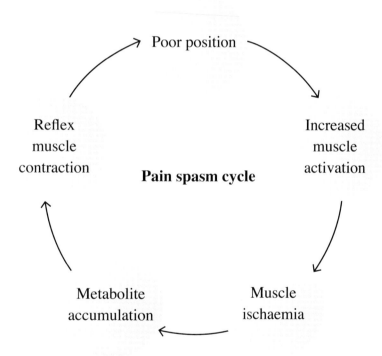

Figure 6.13: Pain spasm model.

Dowager's Hump

It has also been shown that for every inch that the head moves forwards, the compressive forces exerted by the head onto the lower cervical spine are increased by 100% (Calliet, 2003). This creates traction on the posterior ligamentous system of the spine as T1 is pulled into flexion and C7 into relative extension, and the joint space is increased between T1 and T2. As the condition becomes chronic and the cervical spine migrates forwards, extra fat tissue is laid down in an attempt to stabilise the upper thoracic/lower cervical spine. This is commonly known as Dowager's hump.

Upper Body

7

The following upper body muscles will be tested and treated:

- Upper trapezius
- Levator scapulae
- Sternocleidomastoid
- Scalenes
- Latissimus dorsi
- Pectoralis major
- Pectoralis minor
- Coracoid muscles: Biceps brachii short head, coracobrachialis
- Subscapularis
- Infraspinatus

POSTURAL ASSESSMENT SHEET – UPPER BODY

Patient Name:

Key: E = Equal

L/R = Short on left or right side

Muscles	Date:	Date:	Date:
Upper trapezius			
Levator scapulae			
Sternocleidomastoid			
Scalenes			
Latissimus dorsi			
Pectoralis major			
Pectoralis minor			
Coracoid muscles Biceps brachii short head Coracobrachialis			
Subscapularis			
Infraspinatus			

Upper Trapezius

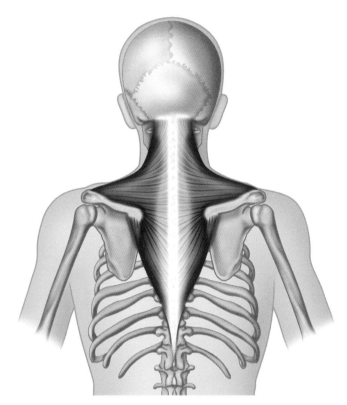

Origin

Base of skull (occipital bone). Spinous processes of seventh cervical vertebra (C7) and all thoracic vertebrae (T1-T12).

Insertion

Lateral third of clavicle. Acromion process. Spine of scapula.

Action

Upper fibres: Pull the shoulder girdle up (elevation). Help prevent depression of the shoulder girdle when a weight is carried on the shoulder or in the hand.
Middle fibres: Retract (adduct) scapula.
Lower fibres: Depress scapula, particularly against resistance, as when using the hands to get up from a chair.
Upper and lower fibres together: Rotate scapula, as in elevating the arm above the head.

Nerve

Accessory X1 nerve. Ventral ramus of cervical nerves (C2, C3, C4).

Assessment of Upper Trapezius

The patient is in a sitting position for this test (figure 7.1). The therapist passively side bends the patient's neck to the right while palpating the left trapezius with their left hand (figure 7.2). The therapist needs to be aware of the bind of the tissue, rather than the patient saying that they feel a stretch. The bind is where the 'slack' is taken out of the tissue before the position of stretch is achieved – it is very important to understand this process of bind as opposed to stretch.

If a range of motion of 45 degrees is achieved, a normal length of trapezius is noted. The test is repeated on the contralateral side for comparison.

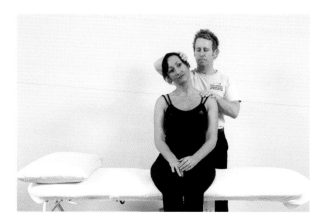

Figure 7.1: Sitting position for upper trapezius assessment.

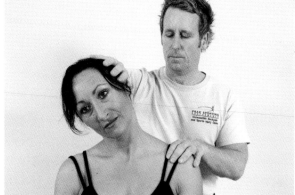

Figure 7.2: The therapist bends the patient's head to the right while stabilising the patient's shoulder with the hand.

Alternative Assessment of Trapezius

Scapula Humeral Rhythm Test

The patient is asked to abduct the right shoulder and the movement is observed. The first 30 degrees of motion comes purely from the glenohumeral joint; after 30 degrees, the scapula starts to rotate. The ratio is generally 2:1 – that is, for every 2 degrees of motion from the glenohumeral joint, there is 1 degree of scapula rotation. For example, at 90 degrees of abduction, 60 degrees would have been performed by the glenohumeral joint and 30 degrees of scapula rotation.

A normal scapula humeral rhythm is shown in figure 7.3, whereas figure 7.4 indicates a 'reverse' scapula humeral rhythm pattern of motion, as the 'upper trapezius' on the right is seen to be overactive and assisting the motion of shoulder abduction. This altered rhythm can be seen very clearly with a condition called adhesive capsulitis or frozen shoulder.

This limited range of motion is due to restricted movement of the glenohumeral joint that can be caused by adhesive capsulitis; the scapula will be the joint of compensation and will be seen to elevate and rotate excessively.

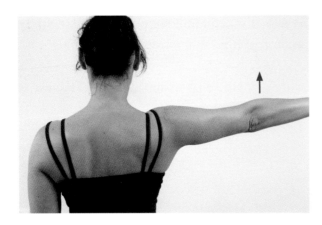

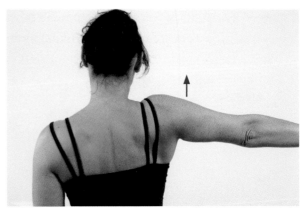

Figure 7.3: Arm abduction – normal scapula humeral rhythm.

Figure 7.4: Arm abduction – reverse scapula humeral rhythm.

Scapula Humeral Rhythm Test With Palpation

To confirm the activation or possibly the overactivation of the upper trapezius during the motion of shoulder abduction, the therapist can place their left hand over the patient's right trapezius while the patient performs the movement (figure 7.5). The therapist notes when they feel the upper trapezius contract. If the contraction is felt within the first 30 degrees of shoulder abduction, the upper trapezius will be classified as overactive.

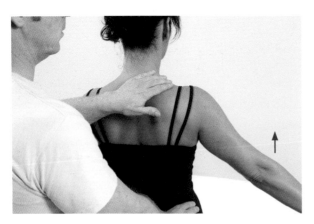

Figure 7.5: The patient abducts their right arm as the therapist palpates the upper trapezius for overactivation.

Assessment of Upper Trapezius From a Supine Position

Patient adopts a supine position with their knees bent, as this helps relax the lumbar spine (figure 7.6). Sitting at the cephalic end of the couch, the therapist places their left hand to cradle the patient's occipital bone and their right hand on top of the patient's right shoulder. Slowly, the therapist passively side bends the patient's head to the left while stabilising the motion from the right shoulder. When the therapist feels the bind from the right upper trapezius, a measurement is taken. A value less than 45 degrees would be classified as short.

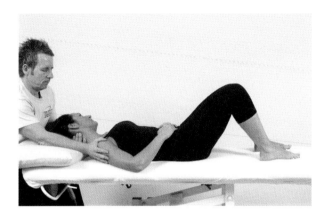

Figure 7.6: Assessment of the upper trapezius from a supine position.

MET Treatment of Right Upper Trapezius

The therapist places the right upper trapezius in a position of bind, and asks the patient to either side bend the cervical spine to the right or elevate the right shoulder. Alternatively, the patient may be requested to perform both of these actions at the same time against a resistance from the therapist. Another way of communicating the technique is to ask the patient to bring the ear to the shoulder, or the shoulder to the ear, against a resistance, holding for 10 seconds.

After the 10-second contraction, the patient is asked to relax, take a breath in and on the relaxation phase the cervical spine is taken further into a left side bend. If the side bending causes any discomfort, the shoulder can be taken into further depression, as this will also have the effect of lengthening the upper trapezius.

If an RI technique is desired, the therapist takes complete control of the patient's cervical spine and shoulder as described above. From this position the patient is asked to reach slowly towards their lower right leg with their right hand, until a point of bind is felt. This approach will activate the lower trapezius as the patient is causing a depression of the right shoulder girdle. This will induce an inhibition of the right upper trapezius, allowing a safe way of lengthening as it will override the activation of the muscle spindles.

The upper trapezius has three fibre components: anterior, medial and posterior. If you decided that certain fibres were tight, a simple rotation of the cervical spine would target specific fibres. Figure 7.7 shows the patient's cervical spine in a half rotation to the left; this targets the middle fibres of the upper trapezius. If you were to take the cervical spine into full rotation, this would target the posterior fibres as seen in figure 7.8. No rotation of the cervical spine would target the anterior fibres.

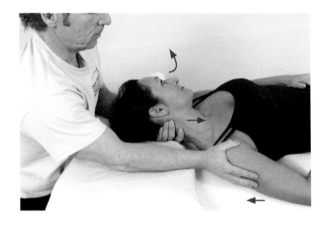

Figure 7.7: The patient is asked to side bend to the right or elevate the right shoulder, or both. Half rotation of the cervical spine emphasises the middle fibres of the trapezius.

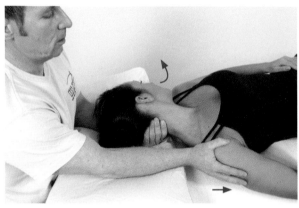

Figure 7.8: The therapist lengthens the right trapezius by applying caudal pressure. Full rotation of the cervical spine emphasises the posterior fibres.

An alternative hand position for the treatment of the upper trapezius is illustrated in figure 7.9. As seen in figures 7.7 and 7.8, the therapist uses a cradle type of hold with their left hand; figure 7.9, however, demonstrates a different hand contact with the therapist using their left hand. Some patients find this position more comfortable.

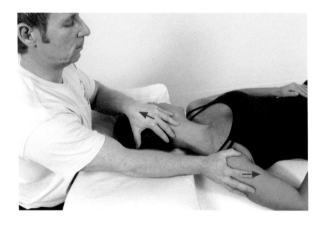

Figure 7.9: An alternative hand position for the treatment of the upper trapezius.

TIP: The upper trapezius often develops trigger points that can be responsible for headaches.

Levator Scapulae

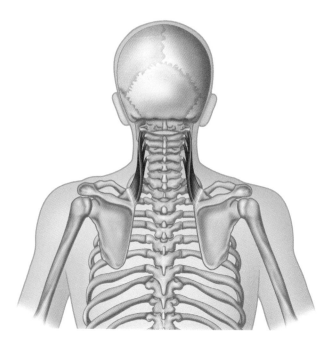

Origin

Transverse processes of the first three or four cervical vertebrae (C1-C4).

Insertion

Upper medial (vertebral) border of the scapula (i.e. portion above the spine of the scapula).

Action

Elevates scapula. Helps retract scapula. Helps bend neck laterally.

Nerve

Dorsal scapular nerve (C4, C5) and cervical nerves (C3, C4).

Assessment of Levator Scapulae

This test for the levator scapulae is very similar to the testing of the upper trapezius. Also, the muscles mentioned have a similar action, i.e. both can elevate the shoulder girdle and side bend the cervical spine. One difference between them is that the upper trapezius assists the upward rotation of the scapula, whereas the levator scapulae assists in downward rotation of the scapulae.

One method of testing the levator scapulae is from the seated position shown in figure 7.10. The therapist gently assists the motion of the head and controls the cervical spine into approximately 30 degrees of right rotation. Once the cervical spine is in the position of rotation, the therapist then encourages cervical flexion and will try to approximate the patient's chin onto their chest. The therapist's right hand prevents the scapula from elevating. When the therapist feels a bind, the range of motion is noted. If the chin can approximate the chest with no resistance, the levator scapulae is classified as normal.

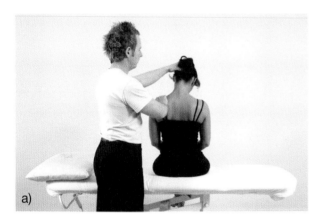 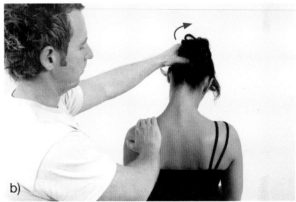

Figure 7.10: (a) Hand positions for assessment of left levator scapulae; (b) Close-up view of hand positions, with the therapist stabilising the shoulder.

MET Treatment of Levator Scapulae

For this treatment the patient is supine. The therapist, while providing support, guides the patient's head into a side bend, followed by flexion. If a resistance is felt prior to the chin touching the chest, this indicates relative shortness of the levator scapulae.

Some therapists find it more appropriate to treat levator scapulae from the test position, rather than placing the patient in an alternative position. It will be a matter of choice, but in my opinion it is generally more comfortable to treat the levator scapulae from the supine position. However, there will be certain times when the patient is unable to adopt a supine position, as this can cause discomfort in some patients who present with cervical spine pain. In this case the seated position would be more appropriate for an MET treatment.

MET treatment of the levator scapulae from the supine position will be described. The hand positioning is similar to that for treatment of the upper trapezius, the difference being that the patient's cervical spine is held more into flexion to achieve the position of bind. This is achieved by the therapist adopting a standing posture rather than a sitting posture (figure 7.11). Standing is preferred since the head may be too heavy to control from the sitting position by using only the arms.

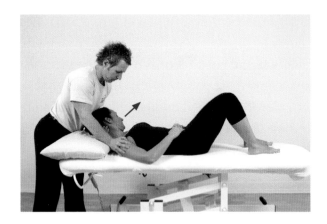

Figure 7.11: Position for MET treatment of levator scapulae.

From the position of bind, the patient is asked to push their cervical spine into extension to initiate the contraction of the levator scapulae. After the appropriate time and on the relaxation, the patient's cervical spine is taken into further flexion, with an added left rotational movement (figure 7.12).

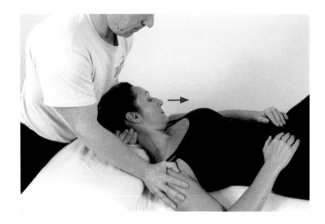

Figure 7.12: The cervical spine is encouraged into further flexion to lengthen the right levator scapulae. The chin is taken towards the chest, with the therapist stabilising the right scapula.

TIP: The levator scapula is working in an eccentric contraction when the cervical position is held in a forward head posture; this indicates that the muscle is in a lengthened position but still in a contracted state. The patient may experience pain at the insertion of the levator scapulae on the superior angle of the scapulae. If this is the case, an MET to lengthen an already lengthened structure might not be appropriate.

Sternocleidomastoid (SCM)

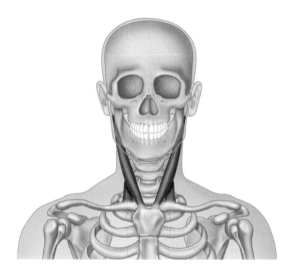

Origin

Sternal head: Anterior surface of upper sternum.
Clavicular head: Medial third of clavicle.

Insertion

Mastoid process of temporal bone (bony prominence just behind the ear).

Action

Contraction of both sides together: Flexes neck (draws head forwards). Raises sternum, and consequently the ribs, during deep inhalation.
Contraction of one side: Tilts the head towards the same side. Rotates head to face the opposite side (and also upwards as it does so).

Nerve

Accessory X1 nerve, with sensory supply for proprioception from cervical nerves (C2, C3).

Assessment of Sternocleidomastoid

The patient is asked to adopt a supine position, knees bent and arms placed by their sides. They are then asked to perform a curl-up from the supine position. The therapist observes the position of the chin and the forehead as the patient performs the curl-up. Figure 7.13 indicates a normal SCM as demonstrated by the forehead leading in a curl-up exercise. Here, the patient has the ability to hold the chin tucked while flexing the trunk.

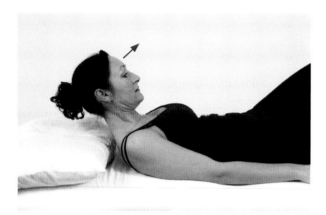

Figure 7.13: The forehead is leading the movement – normal SCM.

If the chin pokes forwards while attempting a curl-up, i.e. the chin leads the movement, the SCM is classified as shortened (figure 7.14).

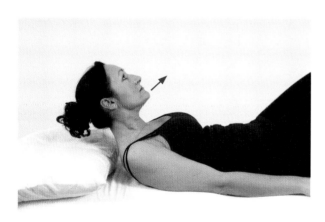

Figure 7.14: The chin leads the movement – shortened SCM.

MET Treatment of Right Sternocleidomastoid

The patient is asked to adopt a supine position, with their knees bent. Having placed a pillow between the patient's shoulder blades, the therapist gently rotates the patient's cervical spine into full left rotation (figure 7.15).

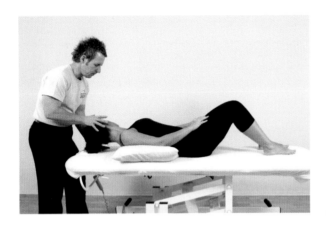

Figure 7.15: MET treatment of right sternocleidomastoid.

The patient is asked to hold this position for about 10 seconds. You can see in figure 7.16 that the patient is holding their head on their own with no involvement from the therapist.

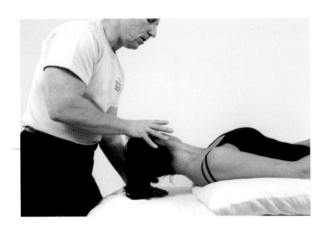

Figure 7.16: The therapist has no contact with the patient's head as the patient is isometrically contracting their right SCM.

Once the patient has isometrically contracted the SCM muscle by holding their head in the rotated position for 10 seconds, the therapist then controls the position of the head, slowly lowering it down onto the couch (figure 7.17a). In some cases, this will already have started to lengthen the SCM.

To achieve an effective lengthening of the right SCM, the therapist places their right hand on the patient's temporal bone and their left hand on the patient's sternum (for females, the patient's hand is placed on their sternum, then the therapist's hand is applied on top). The patient is asked to breathe in, and on the relaxation phase the therapist encourages caudal pressure to their left hand while the right hand stabilises the head (figure 7.17b).

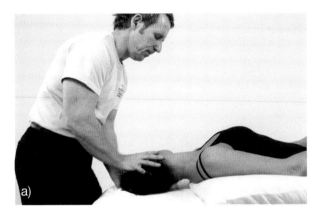 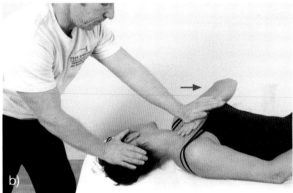

Figure 7.17: a) Therapist is controlling the lowering of the patient's head towards the couch; a) and b) Pressure is applied in a caudal direction with the left hand, while the head is stabilised with the right hand.

TIP: Bilateral contraction of the SCM will give the appearance of a forward head posture. Unilateral contraction of the SCM can result in torticollis, where the cervical spine flexes and rotates away from the side of contracture.

Scalenes

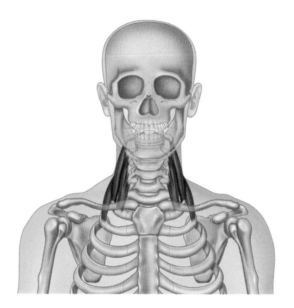

Origin
Transverse processes of cervical vertebrae.

Insertion
Anterior and medius: First rib.
Posterior: Second rib.

Action
Acting together: Flex neck. Raise first rib during a strong inhalation.
Individually: Laterally flex and rotate neck.

Nerve
Ventral rami of cervical nerves (C3-C8).

Assessment of Scalenes

To assess the shortness of the scalenes, one must be aware of the position of the cervical spine and its relationship to the vertebral arteries.

> **Important note: The test that I am about to describe puts the cervical spine into an extended and rotated position. When you are performing the test, if you notice anything strange about the movements of your patient's eyes, or if the patient feels strange or even faint, then you must stop the test immediately, as the vertebral artery is being compromised. If the test demonstrates a positive result for compression of the vertebral artery, you must avoid taking the cervical spine into an extended and rotated position. A safer approach for the treatment of the cervical spine using METs will be from a more flexed position. If you are still unsure, seek the advice of a qualified medical practitioner.**

Assessment of the Right Scalenes

The patient is asked to adopt a supine position, with their knees bent and their head off the end of the couch. The therapist controls the position of the head and gently takes the patient's cervical spine into an extended position (figure 7.18), followed by a side bend to the left and a rotation to the right (figure 7.19).

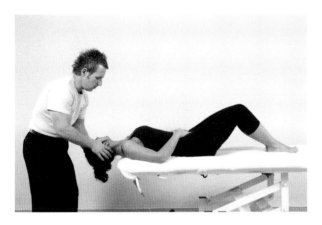

Figure 7.18: Controlling the position of the head, the therapist gently takes the patient's cervical spine into an extended position.

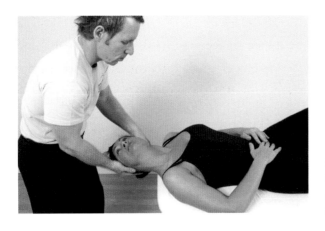

Figure 7.19: From the extended position, the therapist gently takes the patient's cervical spine into a side bend to the left and a rotation to the right.

See figure 7.19 for how to test the tightness of the right scalene. Full rotation of approximately 80 degrees should be achieved. If there is a bind before the full rotation is achieved, the right scalenes are classified as tight.

Another way of looking at the specific tightness of the scalenes; the therapist supports the head and gently takes the cervical spine into extension, a side bend to the right, then rotation to the left (to test the left side); or into extension, a side bend to the left, then rotation to the right (to test the right side). A feeling of resistance prior to full rotation (80 degrees) indicates hypertonicity.

Observation Test for the Relative Shortness of the Scalene Muscle Group

The scalenes are accessory muscles for inspiration. To identify relative shortness, the therapist can observe the respiration cycle with the patient in a supine position (figure 7.20).

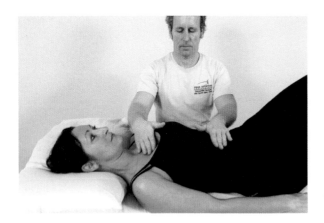

Figure 7.20: The patient lies in a supine position while the therapist observes the respiration cycle.

The patient is asked to breathe in and out normally while the therapist lightly palpates the sternum with their right hand and the area of the diaphragm with their left hand. On the inspiration phase, the therapist observes and feels for motion. If the upper chest is seen to move prior to the diaphragm on inspiration, this indicates possible dysfunction and overactivity of the scalenes.

MET Treatment of Right Scalenes

The patient adopts a position that is very similar to that for treatment of the SCM. A pillow is placed under their shoulder blades and their cervical spine is controlled by the therapist into full left rotation. (The SCM would also be influenced during the treatment of the scalenes.)

The therapist's right hand is placed over the patient's right temporal bone, and the patient's left hand is placed over their left clavicle. The therapist places their left hand on top of the patient's hand.

The patient is asked to breathe in, and the therapist resists the movement from the upper rib cage. The therapist stabilises the position of the patient's head while applying pressure in a caudal direction; this will influence the posterior fibres of the scalene (figure 7.21).

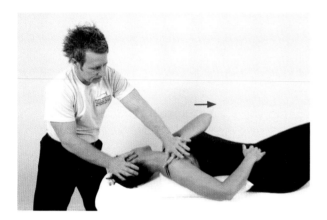

Figure 7.21: MET treatment of right scalenes – posterior fibres.

After the patient has held the full contraction period and on the relaxing exhalation, the therapist applies a caudal pressure to the patient's left hand, which will induce a lengthening of the right scalenes (figure 7.22).

Note: To achieve a lengthening of the scalenes, it is important that the pressure from the therapist is applied on the exhalation, as this also causes a depression of the rib cage.

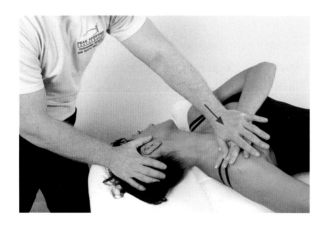

Figure 7.22: Pressure is applied laterally and caudally, with the right hand stabilising the head.

If you are aware of your anatomical origins and insertions, you will know that the scalenes comprise three groups of fibres, similar to the upper trapezius as explained earlier in this chapter.

Due to the anatomical attachments of the scalenes, it is possible to apply a specific technique to influence the lengthening of individual fibres. If you wanted to achieve a lengthening of the posterior fibres of the scalenes, the technique as demonstrated in figure 7.21 can be performed. The technique for lengthening the middle fibres is demonstrated in figure 7.23.

The MET technique shown in figure 7.21, in which the patient has the neck in a full rotation, will influence the posterior fibre of the scalenes. As the insertion of the posterior fibres is on the second rib, the hand position needs to be slightly adjusted. The hand placement is on the second rib, just below the centre of the clavicle.

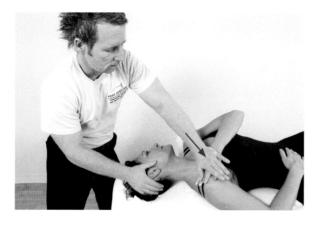

Figure 7.23 demonstrates an MET for the middle fibres of the scalenes, where the cervical spine is rotated midway. If you felt that the anterior fibres of the scalenes needed an MET, the same technique and position would be used, except that there is no rotation of the cervical spine.

TIP: Overactivity of the scalenes anterior (scalenus anticus syndrome) can result in thoracic outlet syndrome (TOS). The neurovascular bundle comes from the C5–T1 vertebrae, known as the brachial plexus, and passes through the fibres of the anterior and middle scalenes, to connect with the subclavian artery. This bundle then continues under the clavicle, over the first rib and under the pectoralis minor. Any compression of the neurovascular bundle can result in pain or altered sensations in the arm and hand.

Latissimus Dorsi

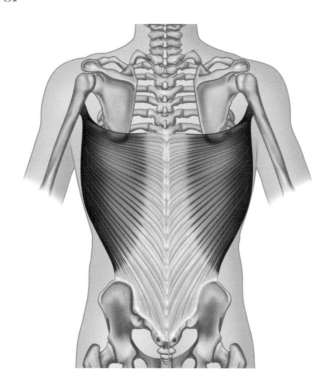

Origin
A broad sheet of tendon which is attached to the spinous processes of lower six thoracic vertebrae and all the lumbar and sacral vertebrae, (T7-S5). Posterior part of iliac crest. Lower three or four ribs. Inferior angle of the scapula.

Insertion
Twists to insert in the intertubercular sulcus (bicipital groove) of the humerus, just below the shoulder joint.

Action
Extends the flexed arm. Adducts and medially rotates the humerus (i.e. draws the arm back and inwards towards the body).
One of the chief climbing muscles, since it pulls the shoulders downwards and backwards, and pulls the trunk up to the fixed arms (therefore also active in crawl swimming stroke).
Assists in forced inspiration, by raising the lower ribs.

Nerve
Thoracodorsal nerve (C6, C7, C8), from the posterior cord of the brachial plexus.

Assessment of Latissimus Dorsi

Arm Elevation Test

To assess tightness of the latissimus dorsi, we can perform a manoeuvre known as the arm elevation test. The therapist slowly takes the patient's arms over their head and tries to sense if there is any bind and the arm wants to adduct (figure 7.24).

It can be seen in figure 7.25 that the patient's right arm is held in a position of adduction, as compared to the left side. You will also notice that the patient's right elbow is flexed; this also indicates a tightness of their right latissimus dorsi.

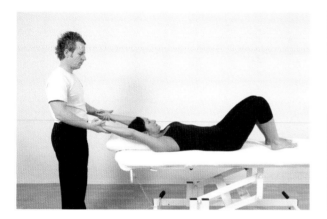

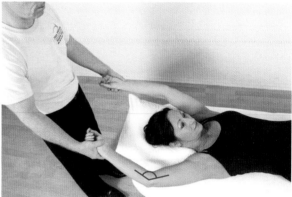

Figure 7.24: Arm elevation test.

Figure 7.25: Tightness of the right latissimus dorsi is indicated.

Alternative Assessment for Latissimus Dorsi

The therapist controls the patient's right arm into an abducted position, and while doing so senses for bind of the latissimus dorsi. To confirm any tightness, the arm is allowed to slightly adduct away from the midline.

From the adducted position of the arm, the therapist tries to straighten the elbow (figure 7.26). If the latissimus dorsi is tight, the arm will be seen to come back to the original position of adduction, confirming that the muscle is held in a shortened position (figure 7.27).

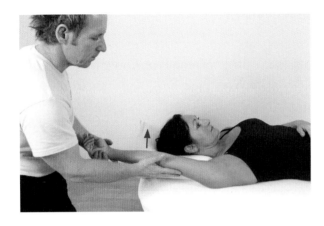

Figure 7.26: The therapist applies pressure to straighten the elbow.

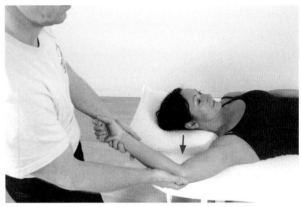

Figure 7.27: The patient's arm deviates laterally due to shortness of the right latissimus dorsi.

MET Treatment of Right Latissimus Dorsi

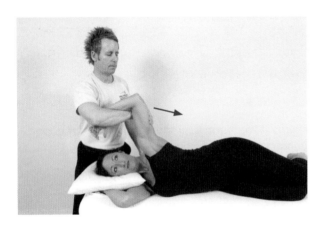

Figure 7.28: The patient pulls their left arm towards the lumbar spine.

The patient lies on their right side and the therapist interlocks their right hand through the patient's left arm. The patient is asked to adduct their left arm to the lumbar spine (figure 7.28). After 10 seconds and on the relaxation phase, the therapist applies pressure to the patient's left iliac crest, as shown in figure 7.29.

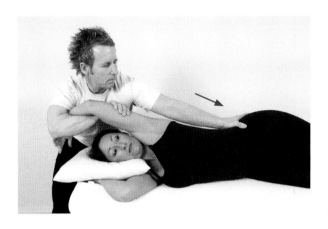

Figure 7.29: Pressure is applied in the direction shown by the arrow to lengthen the left latissimus dorsi. The left hand of the therapist stabilises the iliac crest.

With their left hand, the therapist applies pressure to the patient's left iliac crest. After the contraction, the therapist takes the patient's arm into further abduction; this will lengthen the shortened latissimus dorsi on the left side.

Note: If there is an underlying shoulder pathology – such as acromioclavicular sprain, impingement syndromes or adhesive capsulitis – the technique cannot be performed from this position, as it will generally exacerbate the presenting injury.

TIP: Overactivity, with resultant shortening of the latissimus dorsi, can be a result of gluteus maximus weakness on the contralateral side, due to the relationship of the posterior oblique sling through the thoracolumbar fascia.

Pectoralis Major

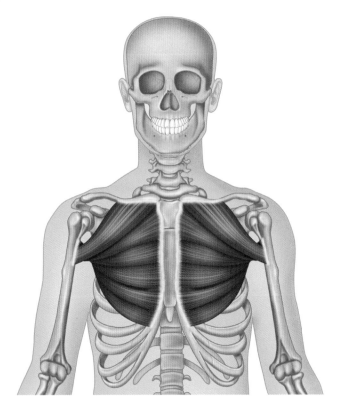

Origin

Clavicular head: Medial half or two-thirds of front of clavicle.

Sternocostal portion: Sternum and adjacent upper six costal cartilages.

Insertion

Upper shaft of humerus.

Action

Adducts and medially rotates the humerus.

Clavicular portion: Flexes and medially rotates the shoulder joint, and horizontally adducts the humerus towards the opposite shoulder.

Sternocostal portion: Obliquely adducts the humerus towards the opposite hip.

One of the main climbing muscles, pulling the body up to the fixed arm.

Nerve

Nerve to upper fibres: Lateral pectoral nerve (C5, C6, C7).

Nerve to lower fibres: Lateral and medial pectoral nerves (C6, C7, C8, T1).

Assessment of Pectoralis Major

Arm Elevation Test

This test is similar to the one that was described for the assessment of the latissimus dorsi, the major difference being the position of the patient's arms. The therapist supports the patient's arms in a fully flexed position, then slowly lowers them towards the couch. If the arms are unable to contact the couch when lowered, one can assume a shortness condition of the pectoralis major.

Figure 7.30 demonstrates the test and indicates that the right and left sides appear to be tight since neither arm is touching the couch. If you look closely, you will see the patient's left arm is held higher off the couch than the right side, which indicates that the left side is the tighter structure. However, you should also note that the right side is tight as well.

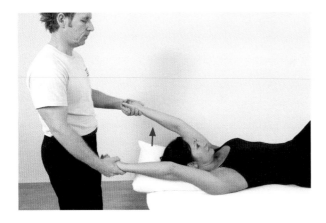

Figure 7.30: The left arm is seen to be higher, compared to the right side.

MET Treatment of Pectoralis Major

In figure 7.31 the therapist is demonstrating the palpation of the patient's right sternal fibres of the pectoralis major; they are palpating the muscle for the point of bind before they perform an MET. The arm is taken away from the body into the scapula plane to induce a lengthening of the pectoralis major.

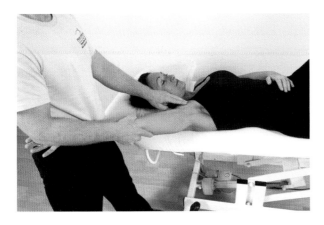

Figure 7.31: The therapist palpates for the point of bind.

From the point of bind, the patient is asked to pull their arm across the body (horizontal flexion) to induce a contraction of the right pectoralis major.

Once the patient has contracted for 10 seconds, the patient (female) is asked to place her hand on her pectoralis major and the therapist places their hand on top of hers. The therapist then controls the patient's right arm and slowly takes the shoulder further away into the scapula plane. This will induce a lengthening of the sternal fibres of the pectoralis major (figure 7.32). Figure 7.33 shows an alternative way of lengthening the pectoralis major for a male patient, in which the therapist applies pressure directly to the pectoralis muscle.

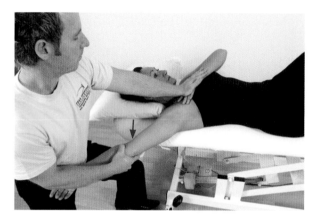

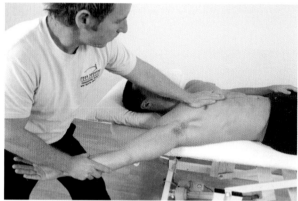

Figure 7.32: The therapist uses their arm to stabilise over the female patient's arm. Pressure is applied in the direction of the left arrow to lengthen the right pectoralis major.

Figure 7.33: An alternative technique for a male patient.

The following technique is used to lengthen the clavicular fibres of the right pectoralis major. The difference in this application as compared to the one described earlier is simply the position of the patient's arm (figure 7.34).

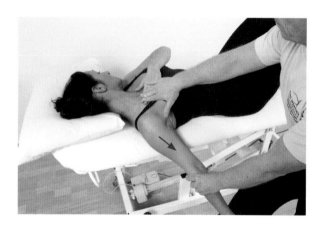

Figure 7.34: Lengthening the clavicular fibres of the pectoralis major. Pressure is applied by the therapist in the direction of the arrow.

The patient's arm is gently taken away from the midline to induce a bind of the clavicular fibres of the right pectoralis major. From the position of bind, the patient is asked to lift their arm against a resistance applied by the therapist. After a 10-second contraction, the clavicular fibres are then taken to their new position of bind.

> *TIP: Protraction of the scapula by the shortening of the pectoralis minor will result in the glenoid fossa rotating medially; this will place the pectoralis major in a shortened position.*

Pectoralis Minor and Coracoid Muscles (Biceps Brachii, Coracobrachialis)

Pectoralis Minor

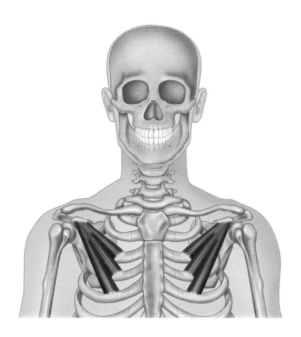

Origin
Outer surfaces of third, fourth and fifth ribs, and fascia of the corresponding intercostal spaces.

Insertion
Coracoid process of scapula.

Action
Draws scapula forwards and downwards. Raises ribs during forced inspiration (i.e. it is an accessory muscle of inspiration if the scapula is stabilised by the rhomboids and trapezius).

Nerve
Medial pectoral nerve with fibres from a communicating branch of the lateral pectoral nerve (C6, C7, C8, T1).

Biceps Brachii

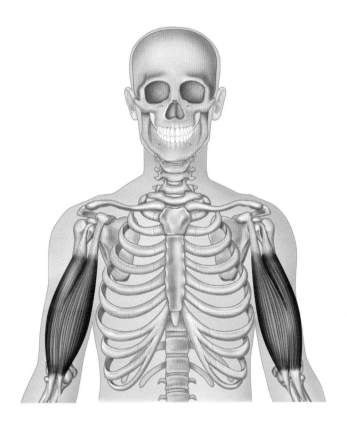

Origin
Short head: Tip of coracoid process of scapula.
Long head: Supraglenoid tubercle of scapula (area just above socket of shoulder joint).

Insertion
Radial tuberosity (on medial aspect of upper part of shaft of radius). Deep fascia (connective tissue) on medial aspect of forearm.

Action
Flexes elbow joint. Supinates forearm. (It has been described as the muscle that puts in the corkscrew and pulls out the cork). Weakly flexes arm at the shoulder joint.

Nerve
Musculocutaneous nerve (C5, C6).

Coracobrachialis

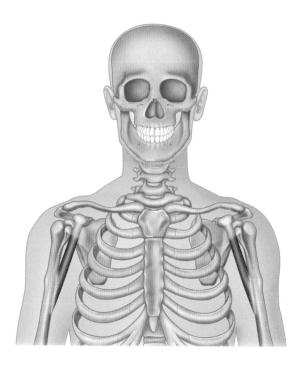

Origin
Tip of coracoid process of scapula.

Insertion
Medial aspect of humerus at mid-shaft.

Action
Weakly adducts shoulder joint. Possibly assists in flexion of the shoulder joint (but this has not been proven). Helps stabilise humerus.

Nerve
Musculocutaneous nerve (C6, C7).

Observational Assessment of Pectoralis Minor

The test for the length of the pectoralis minor is carried out by observation (figure 7.35). The patient is supine as the therapist observes the position of the anterior aspect of the glenohumeral joint. If one shoulder appears to be more anterior, one would suspect a shortened pectoralis minor. (When I refer to the shoulder being anterior, the correct position is where the scapula is protracted.)

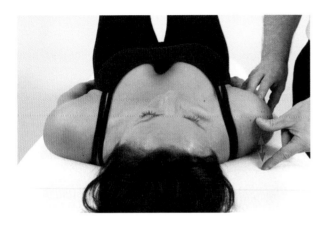

Figure 7.35: Observing the position of the anterior aspect of the glenohumeral joint. The arrow shows that the distance is greater on the right side.

Coracoid Muscles and Differential Diagnosis

Concluding that the relative shortness of the pectoralis minor is responsible for the anterior position, however, might not be correct, as the coracobrachialis and the short head of the biceps brachii also have attachments on the coracoid process.

To try to establish which structure is responsible for the perceived tightness, the therapist controls the patient's right elbow and slowly flexes the elbow (figure 7.36); if the shoulder is seen to return to its neutral position, the biceps brachii short head is the shortened structure.

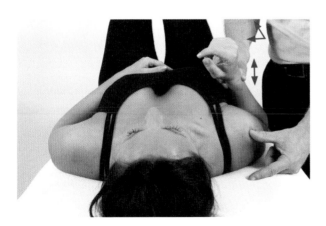

Figure 7.36: Assessment of the short head of the biceps brachii. The elbow is passively flexed and the distance is observed. If it changes, the biceps brachii is short.

Figure 7.37 shows the therapist again cradling the patient's right arm, but this time they are slowly flexing the shoulder. If the shoulder appears to return to the neutral position, the coracobracialis is the muscle that is responsible for the anterior position of the shoulder.

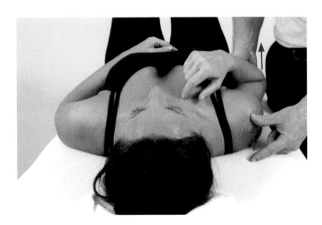

Figure 7.37: Assessment of the coracobracialis. The shoulder is passively flexed and the gap is observed. If it changes, the coracobrachialis is tight.

If neither of these tests is positive then one can assume that the muscle responsible for the position of the shoulder is the pectoralis minor.

MET Treatment of Pectoralis Minor

The patient adopts a supine position and the therapist places their left hand under the patient's right shoulder blade. The therapist then controls the anterior aspect of the patient's right shoulder. The patient is asked to protract the right scapula for the appropriate time (figure 7.38). After the contraction, the therapist encourages the right scapula into a retraction position; this will encourage a lengthening of the right pectoralis minor.

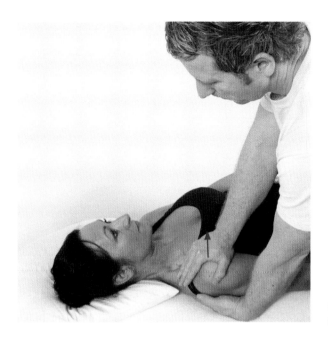

Figure 7.38: The patient protracts their right scapula – supine position.

An alternative MET for the treatment of the pectoralis minor can be performed with the patient in a side-lying position, as seen in figure 7.39. The therapist cradles the patient's right scapula as demonstrated. The patient is asked to protract the right scapula against a resistance applied by the therapist.

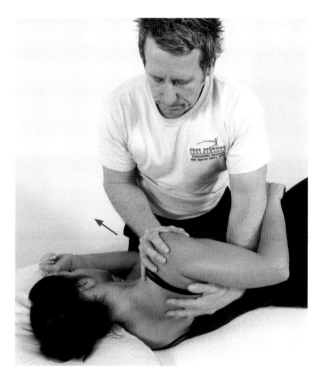

Figure 7.39: The patient protracts their right scapula – side-lying position.

After the 10-second contraction, the therapist gently encourages the right scapula into a retracted position (figure 7.40), which will induce a lengthening of the right pectoralis minor.

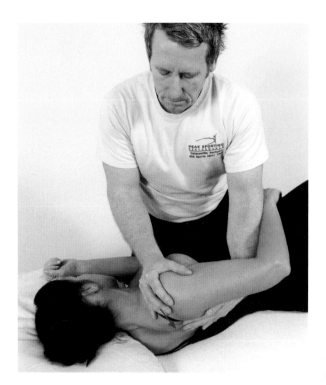

Figure 7.40: The therapist applies a retraction movement to encourage lengthening of the right pectoralis minor.

TIP: The neurovascular bundle travelling from the thoracic outlet contains the brachial plexus and artery. These structures travel underneath the pectoralis minor, so any hypertonicity of this muscle could result in a brachial neuritis or a vascular compromise to the arm/hand.

Subscapularis

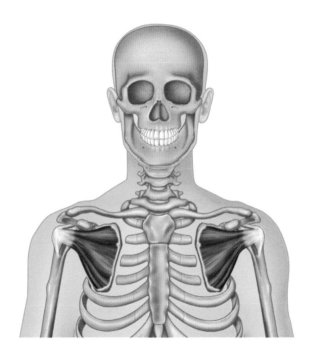

Origin
Subscapular fossa (anterior surface of scapula).

Insertion
Lesser tubercle at the top of humerus. Capsule of shoulder joint.

Action
As a rotator cuff, stabilises shoulder joint; mainly prevents the head of the humerus being pulled upwards by the deltoid, biceps brachii and long head of triceps brachii. Medially rotates humerus.

Nerve
Upper and lower subscapular nerves (C5, C6, C7), from the posterior cord of the brachial plexus.

Assessment of Subscapularis

The therapist takes the patient's arm to 90 degrees of abduction and 90 degrees of elbow flexion – an assessment in this position is known as the 90/90 test. From this position, the therapist supports the patient's elbow with their right hand and the patient's forearm with their left hand (figure 7.41).

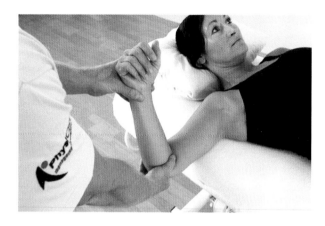

Figure 7.41: Assessment of the subscapularis, starting from the 90/90 position.

The therapist then takes the patient's arm into external rotation until a bind is felt. For normal range of motion of the subscapularis, the external rotation should achieve 90 degrees, i.e. the patient's forearm should be parallel to the couch, as can be seen in figure 7.42(a). If there is shortness of the subscapularis, the range of motion will be less than 90 degrees, as seen in figure 7.42(b).

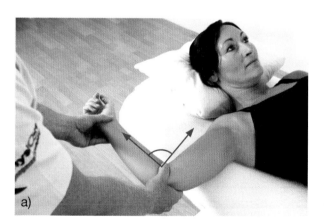 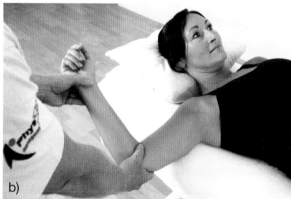

Figure 7.42: (a) The patient's forearm should be parallel to the couch; (b) The subscapularis is held in a shortened position as demonstrated by the limited range of motion in external rotation.

MET Treatment of Subscapularis

PIR Method

The therapist takes the patient's shoulder into external rotation until a bind is felt, as shown in figure 7.43(a). From the position of bind, the patient is asked to contract the subscapularis by internally rotating their shoulder (figure 7.43(b)). After 10 seconds and on the relaxation phase, the therapist applies traction to the shoulder joint (to prevent an impingement) and slowly encourages the shoulder into further external rotation (figure 7.43(c)).

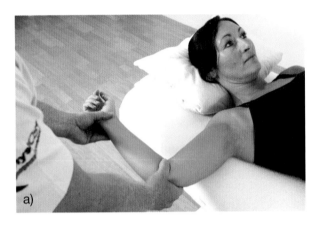
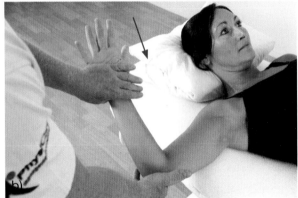

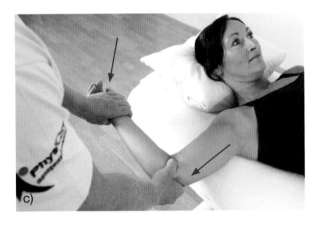

Figure 7.43: MET treatment of the subscapularis – PIR method. (a) Position of bind of the subscapularis; (b) The patient internally rotates the shoulder to activate the subscapularis; (c) After the contraction of the subscapularis, the therapist applies traction to the humerus and encourages further external rotation.

RI Method

If the patient has discomfort activating the subscapularis, the antagonistic muscle of the infraspinatus can be activated instead. From the position of bind (explained above), the patient is asked to resist external rotation; this will contract the infraspinatus and allow the subscapularis to relax through RI. On the relaxation phase, a lengthening procedure of the subscapularis can then be performed.

> TIP: The subscapularis is one of the rotator cuff muscles and is the main medial rotator of the glenohumeral joint. A subscapular strain can result in referred pain to the area of the deltoid tuberosity.

Infraspinatus

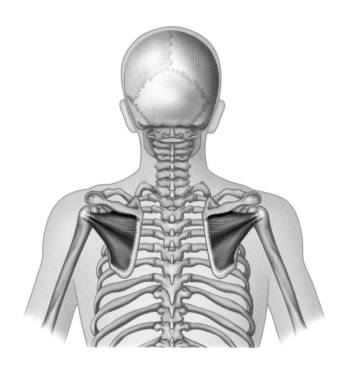

Origin

Middle two-thirds of dorsal surface of scapula, below spine of scapula.

Insertion

Greater tubercle at the top of humerus. Capsule of shoulder joint.

Action

As a rotator cuff muscle, helps prevent posterior dislocation of the shoulder joint. Laterally rotates humerus.

Nerve

Suprascapular nerve (C4, C5, C6), from the upper trunk of the brachial plexus.

Assessment of Infraspinatus

From the 90/90 position, the therapist takes the patient's arm into internal rotation until a bind is felt (figure 7.44(a)). For normal range of motion of the infraspinatus, the internal rotation should achieve 70 degrees, as seen in figure 7.44(b). If the range of motion is less than 70 degrees, the infraspinatus is classified as short.

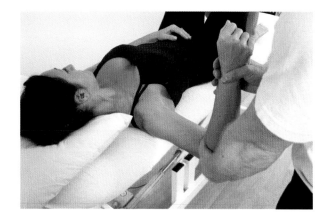
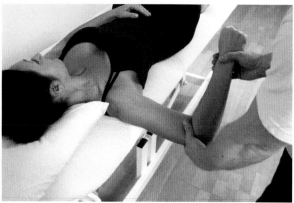

Figure 7.44: (a) Assessment of the infraspinatus from the 90/90 position;

(b) Infraspinatus normal length indicated by the internal rotation achieving 70 degrees.

MET Treatment of Infraspinatus
PIR Method

The therapist takes the shoulder into internal rotation until the position of bind is felt (figure 7.45(a)). From this position, the patient is asked to externally rotate the shoulder (figure 7.45(b)), which will activate the infraspinatus. After the 10-second contraction, the therapist applies traction to the shoulder and slowly encourages the shoulder into further internal rotation (figure 7.45(c)).

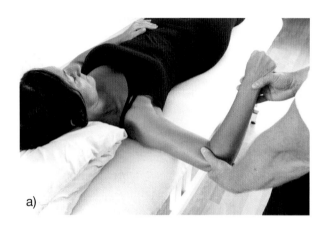

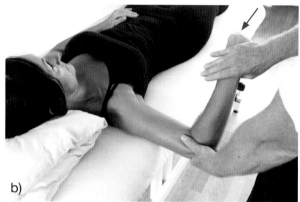

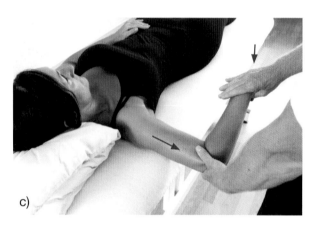

Figure 7.45: MET treatment of the infraspinatus – PIR method. (a) Position of bind for the infraspinatus; (b) The patient is asked to resist external rotation; (c) The therapist applies a traction technique to the humerus and encourages further internal rotation to lengthen the infraspinatus.

RI Method

If the patient has discomfort activating the infraspinatus, the antagonistic muscle of the subscapularis can be activated instead. From the position of bind (explained above), the patient is asked to resist internal rotation. This will contract the subscapularis and allow the infraspinatus to relax through RI. On the relaxation phase, a lengthening procedure of the infraspinatus can then be performed.

> *TIP: Trigger points located within the infraspinatus commonly refer pain to the anterior part of the shoulder.*

Lower Body

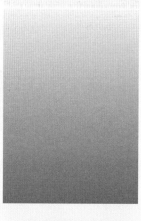

8

The following lower body muscles will be tested and treated:

- Gastrocnemius
- Soleus
- Hamstrings: Semitendinosus, semimembranosus, biceps femoris
- Tensor fasciae latae (TFL) / iliotibial band (ITB)
- Adductors
- Rectus femoris

POSTURAL ASSESSMENT SHEET – LOWER BODY

Patient Name:

Key: E = Equal

          L/R = Short on left or right side

Muscles	Date:	Date:	Date:
Gastrocnemius			
Soleus			
Medial hamstrings			
Lateral hamstrings			
Tensor fasciae latae / iliotibial band			
Adductors			
Rectus femoris			

Gastrocnemius

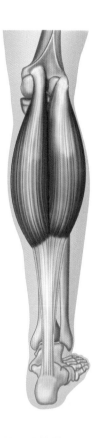

Origin
Medial head: Lower posterior surface of femur above medial condyle.
Lateral head: Lateral condyle and lower posterior surface of femur.

Insertion
Posterior surface of calcaneus (heel bone) via the calcaneal tendon (Achilles tendon), which is a fusion of the tendons of gastrocnemius and soleus.

Action
Plantar flexes (points) foot at ankle joint. Assists in flexion of knee joint. A main propelling force in walking and running.

Nerve
Tibial nerve (S1, S2).

Assessment of Gastrocnemius

The patient's left leg is placed across the therapist's thigh. From this position, the therapist has control of the patient's left lower limb and foot. It is important to make sure that the patient's leg is kept straight at the knee, as this will influence the test result. The therapist gently encourages the patient's left ankle into a dorsiflexed position until a bind is felt (figure 8.1). The normal range of motion should achieve 90 degrees; if the point of bind is felt sooner, the gastrocnemius is classified as short.

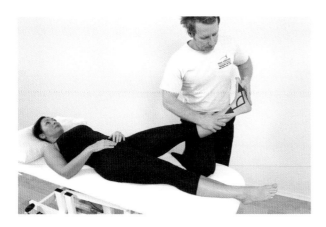

Figure 8.1: The therapist gently encourages the patient's left ankle into a dorsiflexed position until a bind is felt. A range of motion of 90 degrees is normal.

Alternative Method for Testing the Muscle Length of the Gastrocnemius

This test can be performed if the patient has a normal range of motion in their hamstrings; if the hamstrings have been classified as short, the original test described above must be used.

The therapist passively takes the patient's left leg to 90 degrees of hip flexion. From this position, the therapist controls the patient's left lower limb and stabilises the ankle. The therapist slowly encourages the patient's ankle into dorsiflexion and feels for a bind, as shown in figure 8.2; if a range of 90 degrees can be achieved with no resistance, the gastrocnemius is classified as normal.

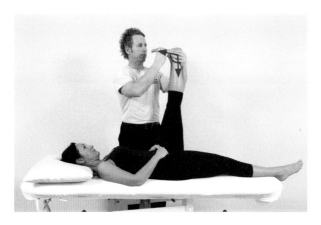

Figure 8.2: Testing the gastrocnemius: a range of motion of 90 degrees is normal. This technique also gives an indication of hamstring length.

MET Treatment of Gastrocnemius

The patient is asked to push their toes away (plantar flexion) to activate the gastrocnemius (figure 8.3(a) and (c)). After a 10-second contraction and on the relaxation phase, the therapist encourages dorsiflexion to promote lengthening of the gastrocnemius (figure 8.3(b) and (d)).

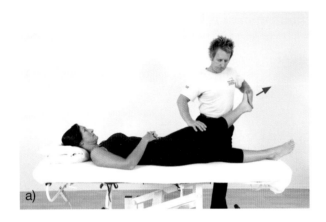 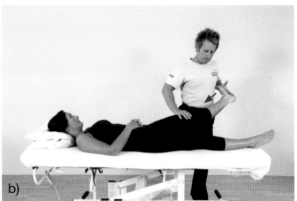

Figure 8.3: (a) Contraction of gastrocnemius; (b) Lengthening of gastrocnemius.

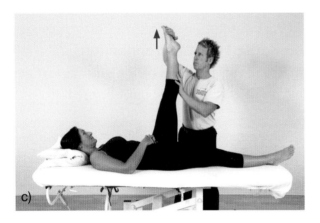 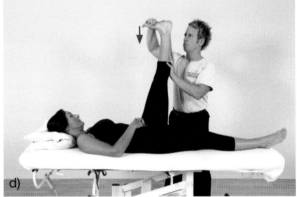

Figure 8.3: (c) The patient plantar flexes the ankle from 90 degrees of hip flexion; (d) After the contraction, the therapist encourages dorsiflexion of the ankle to lengthen the gastrocnemius.

TIP: Common tears of the gastrocnemius occur at the musculotendinous junction (MTJ); in sports medicine this injury is referred to as tennis leg.

Soleus

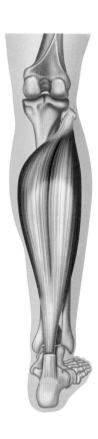

Origin

Upper posterior surfaces of tibia and fibula.

Insertion

With gastrocnemius, via calcaneal tendon, on posterior surface of calcaneus (heel bone).

Action

Plantar flexes ankle joint. The soleus is frequently in contraction during standing to prevent the body falling forwards at the ankle joint, i.e. to offset the line of pull through the body's centre of gravity. Thus, it helps to maintain the upright posture.

Nerve

Tibial nerve (L5, S1, S2).

Assessment of Soleus

This test is similar to the one for the gastrocnemius, the difference being that the patient's knee is flexed – this will relax and slacken the gastrocnemius due to its anatomical attachment on the posterior femoral condyles.

With the knee in slight flexion, the therapist controls the position of the lower limb and ankle, as seen in figure 8.4. From this position, the therapist slowly encourages dorsiflexion of the ankle until a bind is felt. The normal range of motion is 90 degrees; any binding experienced before this indicates shortness in soleus.

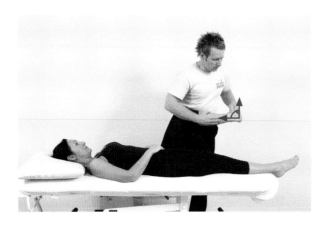

Figure 8.4: The knee is bent to specify the soleus. In this position, the normal range of motion of the ankle is 90 degrees.

MET Treatment of Soleus

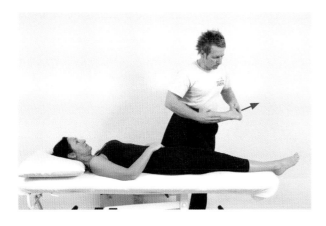

Figure 8.5: The patient plantar flexes the ankle.

From the position of bind, the patient is asked to plantar flex the ankle to activate the contraction in the soleus muscle (figure 8.5). After a 10-second contraction and on the relaxation phase, the therapist gently encourages the ankle into further dorsiflexion as shown in figure 8.6.

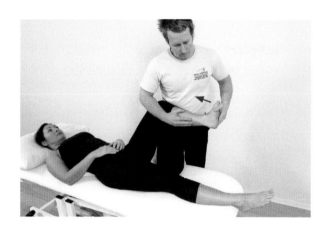

Figure 8.6: The therapist lengthens the soleus by dorsiflexing the ankle.

TIP: The soleus and the gastrocnemius are known as the triceps surae, which relates to three muscles of the lower leg: the two heads of the gastrocnemius and one head of the soleus.

Hamstrings

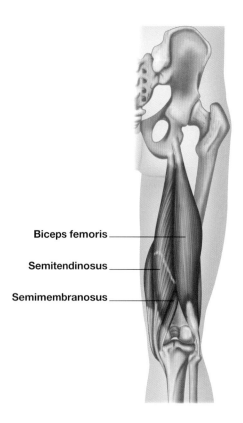

Biceps femoris

Semitendinosus

Semimembranosus

Origin
Ischial tuberosity (sitting bone). Biceps femoris also originates from the back of the femur.

Insertion
Semimembranosus: Back of medial condyle of tibia (upper inside part of tibia).
Semitendinosus: Upper medial surface of shaft of tibia.
Biceps femoris: Head (top) of fibula. Lateral condyle of tibia (upper outside part of tibia).

Action
Flex the knee joint. Extend the hip joint.
Semimembranosus and semitendinosus also medially rotate (turn in) the lower leg when knee is flexed. Biceps femoris laterally rotates (turns out) the lower leg when the knee is flexed.

Nerve
Branches of the sciatic nerve (L4, L5, S1, S2, S3).

General Assessment of Hamstrings

Hip Flexion Test

This test helps to provide the practitioner with an overall impression of the general length of the hamstring muscles. The patient lies in a supine position with both legs extended. The therapist passively guides the patient's left hip into flexion until a point of bind is felt. The normal range is between 80 and 90 degrees; less than 80 degrees indicates that the hamstrings are held in a shortened position. However, 'neural tension' of the sciatic nerve and a specific hamstring injury can also restrict the range of motion of the hip joint.

As you can see in figure 8.7, the patient has a normal range of motion in their hamstrings. Anything less than 80-90 degrees would be classified as short.

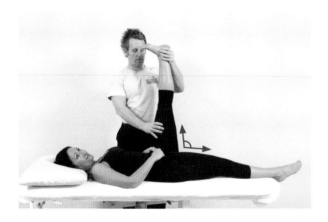

Figure 8.7: Hip flexion test. A range of motion of 80-90 degrees is normal.

MET Treatment of Hamstrings (Non-Specific)

The following technique is very good for lengthening the hamstrings as a group; later on in this chapter we will see how to specifically target the medial and lateral hamstrings.

The therapist adopts a standing posture and passively controls the patient's right leg into hip flexion until a bind is felt in the hamstrings. From this position, the patient's lower leg is placed on the therapist's right shoulder, as shown in figure 8.8.

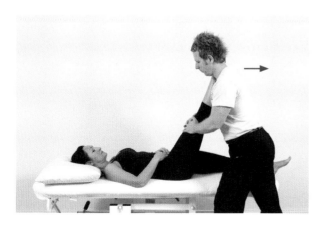

Figure 8.8: The patient pushes their right leg down against the therapist's shoulder.

The patient is asked to push down against the shoulder of the therapist for 10 seconds. After the contraction of the hamstrings and on the relaxation phase, the therapist passively takes the right leg into further flexion, as seen in figure 8.9.

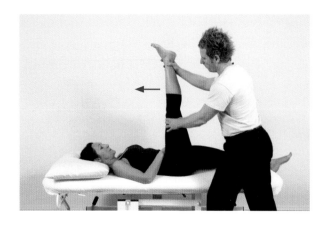

Figure 8.9: The therapist passively takes the hip into further flexion.

Alternative MET for the Insertion of the Hamstrings

This technique is very good for lengthening the insertion aspect of the hamstrings. The patient's hip is now flexed to 90 degrees and the lower leg is placed over the shoulder of the therapist, as shown in figure 8.10.

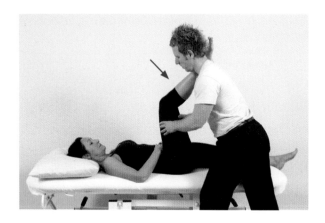

Figure 8.10: With their hip flexed to 90 degrees, the patient's lower leg is placed over the therapist's shoulder.

From this position, the patient is asked to pull their heel towards their gluteal muscles, as this will activate the contraction of the hamstrings. After a 10-second contraction and on the relaxation phase, the therapist passively encourages knee extension until a new point of bind is felt, as shown in figure 8.11.

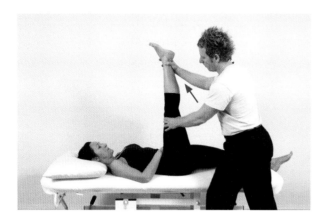

Figure 8.11: The therapist passively encourages knee extension to lengthen the hamstrings.

RI Method

The patient is asked to contact the hamstrings as described above; however, after the 10-second contraction and on the relaxation phase, the patient is asked to slowly straighten their knee (which was flexed to start with) as the therapist passively takes the knee into further extension. The patient will be contracting their quadriceps as they straighten the knee actively; this will induce an RI of the hamstrings, allowing a more effective and safe lengthening to occur.

Assessment of the Medial Hamstrings – Semitendinosus and Semimembranosus

After conducting a general assessment of the hamstrings, if the range of motion is less than 80 degrees, we can conclude that there is a soft tissue restriction present within the hamstring muscle group. However, the assessment does not tell us which aspect of the hamstrings is the tighter structure.

With specific testing it is possible to identify the individual components of the hamstring muscles that are responsible; the testing methods that will be described next allow the therapist to distinguish between the lateral and medial hamstrings.

The following tests can be incorporated into the assessment to help differentiate muscle length anomalies in the medial hamstrings from those in the lateral hamstrings.

In order to investigate whether the semitendinosus or the semimembranosus is the restrictive tissue, the medial hamstrings are isolated as follows. The patient's leg is controlled by the therapist, who applies an external rotation and abduction while the hip is passively flexed (figure 8.12). The point of bind is noted and if the range of motion is less than that in the original test, the medial hamstrings can be assumed to be the shortened muscles.

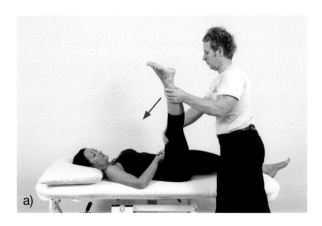

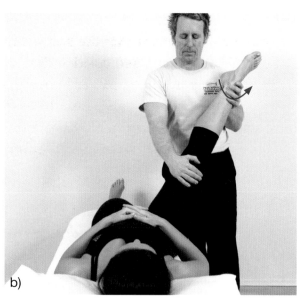

Figure 8.12(a) and (b): To specifically identify the medial hamstrings as the restrictive tissue, the patient's leg is externally rotated and abducted while the hip is passively flexed.

Lateral Hamstrings – Biceps Femoris

This specific test will isolate the biceps femoris. The therapist applies an internal rotation and adduction while the patient's leg is taken into passive flexion (figure 8.13). If the motion feels restrictive, the therapist needs to determine whether the range of motion is less than that in the original hip flexion test. If it is, the lateral hamstring of the biceps femoris can be identified as short.

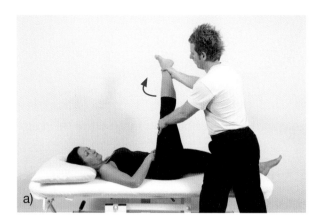

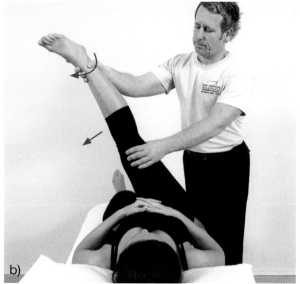

Figure 8.13(a) and (b): The therapist applies an internal rotation and adduction while the leg is taken into passive flexion.

Note: It is important that the hamstrings are treated in a position that is related to the particular sport and position that may have caused the initial trauma. Take, for example, a male rugby player injuring his right hamstring while rotating his trunk to the left to pass the ball. This athlete will need his right hamstring lengthened, and to achieve a specific stretch the hip will need to be taken into a rotation, as explained above, to specifically identify the injured hamstring.

TIP: Remember that the medial and lateral hamstrings might need treating individually rather than together.

Tensor Fasciae Latae (TFL) / Iliotibial Band (ITB)

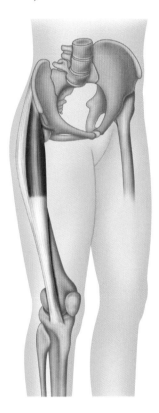

Origin
Outer edge of iliac crest, towards the front.

Insertion
Joins iliotibial tract (long fascia lata tendon) just below the hip, which runs to the upper lateral side of the tibia.

Action
Flexes, abducts and medially rotates hip joint. Tenses the fascia lata, thus stabilising the knee.

Nerve
Superior gluteal nerve (L4, L5, S1).

Assessment of Tensor Fasciae Latae

Ober's Test

This test was first described in 1935 by Frank Ober, who wrote an article called 'Back strain and sciatica'. Ober discussed the relationship of a contracted tensor fasciae latae and the iliotibial band to lower back pain and sciatica.

The patient is asked to adopt a side-lying position, and the therapist (with the assistance of the patient) places the patient's shoulder, hip and knee in alignment as shown in figure 8.14(a).

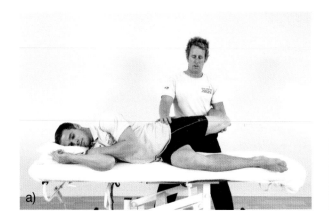
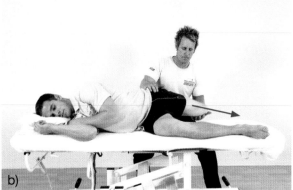
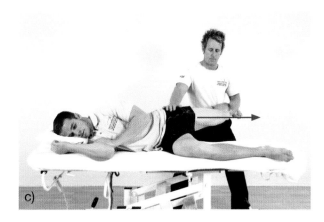
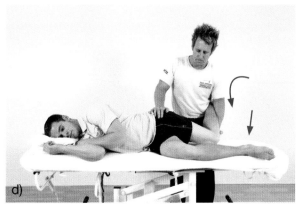

Figure 8.14: Ober's test. (a) The therapist controls the patient's left knee and asks the patient to relax fully before the knee is lowered towards the couch; (b) The knee dropping down indicates a normal length of TFL/ITB; (c) The knee remaining where it is indicates a tight TFL/ITB; (d) The hip is allowed to 'fall' into hip flexion and internal rotation. One could mistakenly consider the TFL/ITB to be normal length, but a 'tight' TFL/ITB will take the hip into this dysfunctional position.

When the therapist feels that the patient has sufficiently relaxed, they slowly bends their own knees (as in a half squat) while maintaining control of the patient's left knee as it is lowered to the couch. If the knee is seen to drop below the level of parallel, the TFL/ITB is classified as normal; if the thigh remains or drops only slightly below parallel, the TFL/ITB is classified as short.

Note: If there is shortness within the tensor fasciae latae and iliotibial band, the leg will remain relatively abducted. It is important to be careful not to allow the hip to fall into internal rotation and hip flexion.

If the tensor fasciae latae and the iliotibial band are held in a shortened position, the hip will want to 'fall' into hip flexion with internal rotation as the therapist lowers the leg. If this is allowed to happen, one could mistakenly assume a 'normal' length of the tensor fasciae latae and iliotibial band as the leg approximates the couch. Therefore, the therapist has to be very diligent when controlling the patient's leg during the test and not allow the hip to flex and internally rotate.

MET Treatment of Tensor Fasciae Latae and Iliotibial Band

The patient adopts a supine position, and the therapist crosses the patient's flexed left leg over their right leg. The therapist controls the patient's left knee with their right hand and holds onto the patient's right ankle with their left hand, as shown in figure 8.15. The patient's right leg is then placed into the adducted position until a bind is felt. From the position of bind, the patient is asked to abduct their right leg against a resistance applied by the therapist.

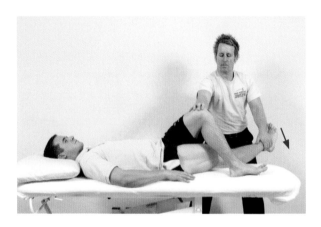

Figure 8.15: The patient abducts their right leg.

After a 10-second contraction and on the relaxation phase, the therapist passively takes the patient's right leg into further adduction (figure 8.16). This will lengthen the right TFL and ITB.

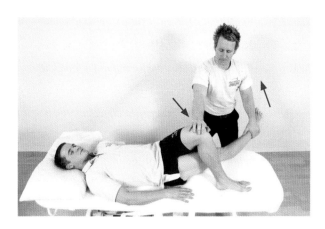

Figure 8.16: The patient's left knee is stabilised while the therapist adducts the right leg.

TIP: Hypertonicity of the tensor fasciae latae can cause an overactivity of the iliotibial band. This can eventually induce a friction syndrome on the lateral femoral condyle of the knee, commonly called runner's knee.

Adductors

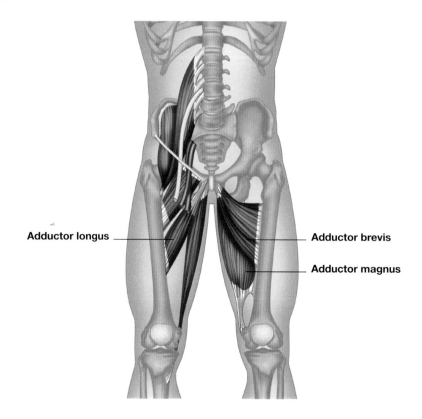

Adductor longus — — Adductor brevis

— Adductor magnus

Origin
Anterior part of pubic bone (ramus). Adductor magnus also has its origin on the ischial tuberosity.

Insertion
Whole length of medial side of femur, from hip to knee.

Action
Adduct and medially rotate hip joint.

Nerve
Magnus: Obturator nerve (L2, L3, L4). Sciatic nerve (L4, L5, S1).
Brevis: Obturator nerve (L2, L3, L4).
Longus: Obturator nerve (L2, L3, L4).

Assessment of Adductors

Hip Abduction Test

The patient adopts a supine position on the couch. The therapist takes hold of the patient's left leg and passively abducts the hip while palpating the adductors with their right hand (figure 8.17). When they feel a bind, the position is noted; the normal range of motion for passive abduction is 45 degrees. If the range is less than this, a tight adductor group is indicated.

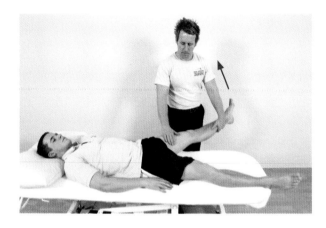

Figure 8.17: The therapist abducts and palpates the adductors for bind.

However, there is an exception to the rule. If the range of motion is less than 45 degrees, it could be that the medial hamstrings are restricting the movement of passive abduction. To differentiate between the short adductors and the medial hamstrings, the knee is flexed to 90 degrees (figure 8.18); if the range now increases, this indicates shortness in the medial hamstrings.

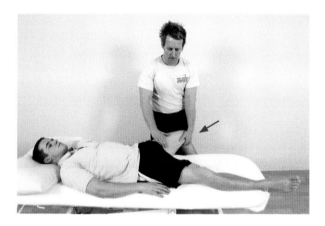

Figure 8.18: The knee is bent to isolate the short adductors.

So to recap, to identify if the hamstrings are the restrictive factor, the therapist passively flexes the knee and then continues with the passive abduction, as shown in figure 8.18. If the range of motion improves, the hamstrings are the restrictive tissues and not the short adductors.

Note: The term short adductors refers to all of the adductor muscles that attach to the femur, the exception being the gracilis. This muscle attaches to a point below the knee, on the pes anserinus area of the medial knee, and acts on the knee as well as the hip.

MET Treatment of Adductors

One of the most effective ways of lengthening the adductors (short) is to utilise an MET from the position that is demonstrated in figure 8.19. The patient adopts a supine position with knees bent and heels together; slowly, the hips are passively taken into abduction by the therapist until a bind is felt in the adductors.

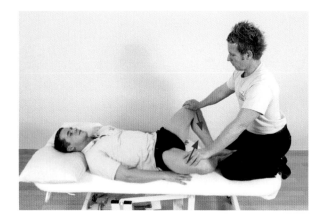

Figure 8.19: The patient adducts their legs.

From the position of bind, the patient is asked to adduct their hips against resistance applied by the therapist, to contract the short adductors. After a 10-second contraction and on the relaxation phase, the hips are then passively taken into further abduction by the control of the therapist (figure 8.20).

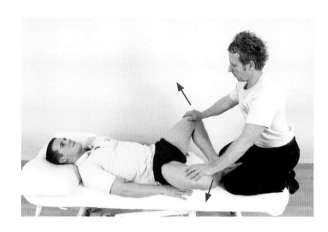

Figure 8.20: The therapist lengthens the adductors.

TIP: Overactivity of the adductors will result in a weakness inhibition of the abductors, in particular the gluteus medius. This can result in a 'Trendelenburg' pattern of gait.

Rectus Femoris

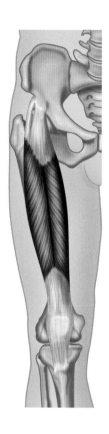

Origin
Straight head (anterior head): Anterior inferior iliac spine.
Reflected head (posterior head): Groove above acetabulum (on ilium).

Insertion
Patella, then via patellar ligament to tuberosity of tibia.

Action
Extends the knee joint and flexes the hip joint (particularly in combination movements, such as in kicking a ball). Assists iliopsoas in flexing the trunk on the thigh. Prevents flexion at knee joint as heel strikes the ground during walking.

Nerve
Femoral nerve (L2, L3, L4).

Assessment of Rectus Femoris

Modified Thomas Test

This test is an excellent way of identifying shortness not only in the rectus femoris but also in the iliopsoas (see Chapter 9). The patient adopts the position as demonstrated in figure 8.21, where they are holding onto their left leg initially, as the right rectus femoris will be tested first.

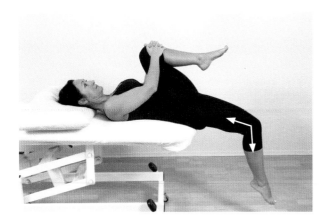

Figure 8.21: To test the right rectus femoris, the patient lies on the couch and holds onto their left leg. A normal length of the rectus femoris is shown.

The patient is asked to pull the left knee towards their chest, as this will posteriorly rotate the innominate on that side; this will be the test position. From this position, the therapist looks at the position of the patient's right knee and right ankle. The angular position of the knee to the ankle should be about 90 degrees; a normal length of the right rectus femoris is shown in figure 8.21.

In figure 8.22, the therapist demonstrates the position of the right knee compared to the right ankle. Here, the lower leg is seen to be held in an extended position, which confirms the tightness of the right rectus femoris.

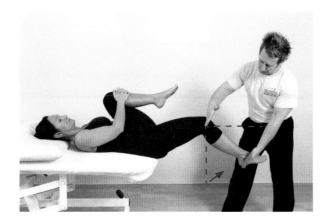

Figure 8.22: The knee is held in extension, indicating a tight rectus femoris.

Note: In figure 8.22 you will also notice the position of the hip – it is held in a flexed position. This indicates a tightness of the iliopsoas and is discussed later in Chapter 9.

MET Treatment of Rectus Femoris

The patient is asked to adopt a prone position, and the therapist passively flexes the patient's right knee until a bind is felt. At the same time, the therapist stabilises the sacrum with their right hand, which will prevent the pelvis from rotating anteriorly and stressing the lower lumbar spine facet joints.

Note: If you consider the patient to have an increased lumbar lordosis, a pillow can be placed under their stomach, as shown in the figure. This will help flatten the lordosis and can help reduce any potential discomfort that they might experience.

From the position of bind, the patient is asked to extend their knee against a resistance applied by the therapist. After a 10 second-contraction and on the relaxation phase, the therapist encourages the knee into further flexion, which will lengthen the rectus femoris, as seen in figure 8.23 and figure 8.24(a) and (b).

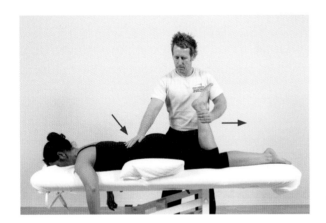

Figure 8.23: The patient extends their knee while the therapist stabilises the lumbar spine.

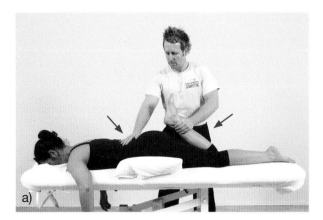

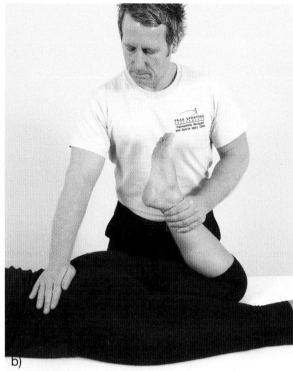

Figure 8.24: (a) The therapist passively flexes the patient's knee to lengthen the rectus femoris while stabilising the lumbar spine; (b) The knee is flexed further.

Figure 8.25 demonstrates a further lengthening at the origin of the rectus femoris. The initial contraction is exactly the same as depicted in figure 8.23. After the contraction and on the relaxation phase, the therapist controls the knee and slowly flexes the knee and hip at the same time. This will induce a lengthening at the origin and at the insertion of the rectus femoris.

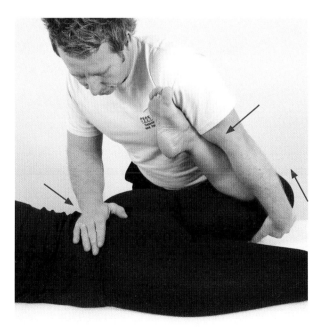

Figure 8.25: The therapist flexes the patient's knee, stabilises the lumbar spine and then extends the hip joint.

Alternative MET Treatment of Rectus Femoris Based On the Modified Thomas Test

Some patients may find that the previous MET for the rectus femoris puts a strain on their lower back. An alternative and possibly a more effective MET for the rectus femoris is based on the modified Thomas test position.

The patient adopts the position of the modified Thomas test as described earlier (page 129). The therapist controls the position of the patient's right thigh and passively flexes their right knee, slowly, towards their bottom. There will be a bind very soon from this position, so take extra care when you are performing this technique for the first time.

From the position of bind, the patient is asked to extend the knee against a resistance applied by the therapist (figure 8.26). After the 10-second contraction and on the relaxation phase, the therapist passively takes the knee into further flexion (figure 8.27). This is a very effective way of lengthening a tight rectus femoris.

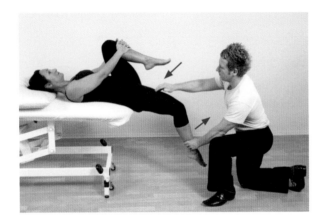

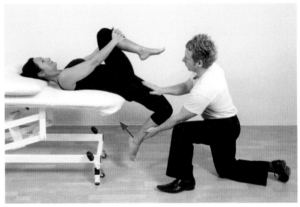

Figure 8.26: The therapist palpates the rectus femoris, and the patient is asked to extend their knee.

Figure 8.27: The therapist passively flexes the knee to lengthen the rectus femoris.

TIP: Bilateral hypertonicity of the rectus femoris will cause the pelvis to adopt an anterior tilt, resulting in lower back pain due to the fifth lumbar vertebra facet joints being forced into a lordotic position.

Trunk / Pelvis and Hip

9

The following muscles of the trunk / pelvis and hip will be tested and treated:

- Piriformis
- Quadratus lumborum (QL)
- Iliopsoas: Psoas major and iliacus
- Erector spinae

POSTURAL ASSESSMENT SHEET – TRUNK / PELVIS AND HIP

Patient Name:

Key: E = Equal

L/R = Short on left or right side

Muscles	Date:	Date:	Date:
Piriformis			
Quadratus lumborum			
Psoas major and iliacus			
Lumbar spine erector spinae			

Piriformis

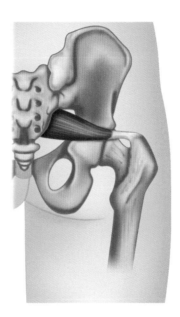

Origin
Internal (front) surface of sacrum.

Insertion
Greater trochanter (top) of femur.

Action
Laterally rotates hip joint. Abducts the thigh when hip is flexed. Helps hold head of femur in its socket.

Nerve
Ventral rami of lumbar nerve (L5) and sacral nerves (S1, S2).

Assessment of Piriformis

The first assessment of the relative length of the piriformis is by observation. The patient is asked to adopt the supine position, and the patient's lower limbs are observed from the cephalic end of the couch. The focus of attention will be on the foot.

As you can see in figure 9.1(a), the patient's left foot appears to be further away from the midline, as compared to the right foot. The actual movement has come from the hip, which is in a position of external rotation. This possibly relates to a tight piriformis on the left side.

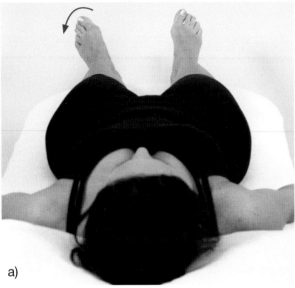

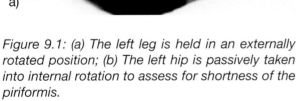

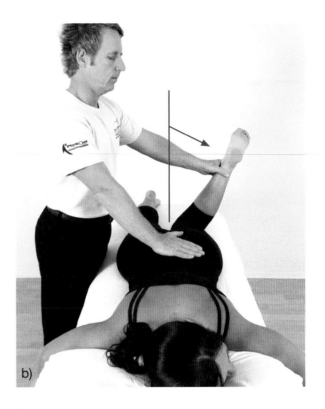

Figure 9.1: (a) The left leg is held in an externally rotated position; (b) The left hip is passively taken into internal rotation to assess for shortness of the piriformis.

Observation Assessment of the Position of the Hip

In order to look at the position of the hip to help us decide whether the piriformis is held in a shortened position, we ask the patient to adopt a prone position. One of the patient's knees is flexed to 90 degrees, and the hip is passively controlled by the therapist and allowed to internally rotate. This is repeated with the other knee flexed to 90 degrees. The side which has the least range of motion indicates relative shortness of the piriformis (figure 9.1(b)).

Another way of assessing the relative length of the piriformis is as follows. The patient is asked to adopt a prone position with both of their knees bent and then to let their legs 'flop out'; this will induce internal rotation of the hip joints.

From the cephalic position of the patient, the therapist observes the position of the lower limb. As you can see in figure 9.2, the lower limb appears to be asymmetric on one side. One can assume that the patient's left side is the dysfunctional side, as the hip is in a position of external rotation. In this case, internal rotation of the hip is restricted, and one can assume that the piriformis on that side is held in a shortened position.

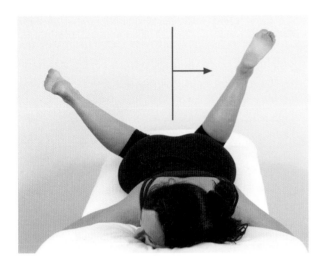

Figure 9.2: A decreased range of motion of the left hip, indicating a tight left piriformis.

MET Treatment of Piriformis

The patient adopts the position of the test as described above, but with the right leg straight and the left knee bent. The therapist makes sure that the pelvis/sacrum is stabilised with their right hand, while controlling the patient's left leg with their left hand. The patient's left leg is passively taken into internal rotation until the position of bind is felt, and the patient is asked to contract the piriformis by pulling their leg against resistance offered by the therapist's left hand. This will induce an external rotation of the hip joint (figure 9.3).

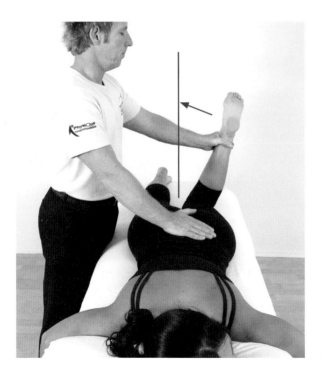

Figure 9.3: The patient pulls their left leg across their body. The therapist stabilises the lumbar spine with the right hand.

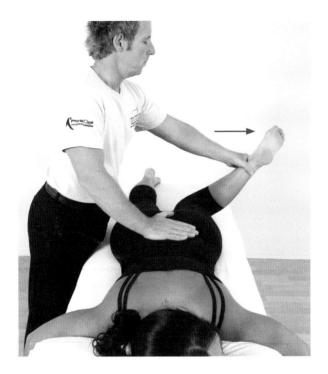

After a 10-second contraction of the piriformis and on the relaxation phase, the therapist takes the patient's left hip into further internal rotation. This will lengthen the piriformis, as shown in figure 9.4.

Figure 9.4: The therapist lengthens the piriformis while stabilising the lumbar spine.

Alternative MET Technique for the Piriformis

This time the patient is asked to adopt a supine position, and the therapist passively takes the patient's left leg and crosses it over the patient's right leg. Controlling the movement of the patient's left innominate with their right hand, the therapist applies pressure to the patient's left knee, passively inducing adduction of the hip to the point of bind (figure 9.5(a)).

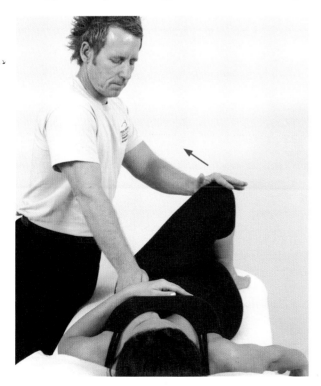

Figure 9.5: (a) The patient abducts their left hip while the therapist stabilises the lumbar spine with the right hand; (b) From the point of bind, the patient abducts against the pressure applied by the therapist in the direction of the arrow.

The patient is asked to abduct their left leg (the piriformis is an abductor) while the therapist resists the movement, as shown in figure 9.5(b). After a 10-second contraction and on the relaxation phase, the therapist passively takes the patient's left leg into further adduction, as shown in figure 9.6.

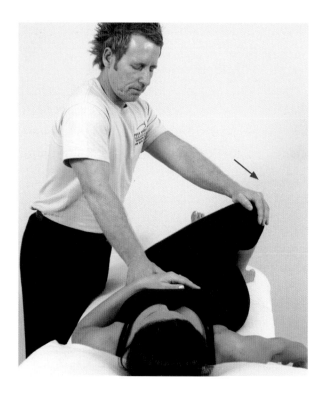

Figure 9.6: The therapist takes the left leg into further adduction and stabilises the lumbar spine with the right hand.

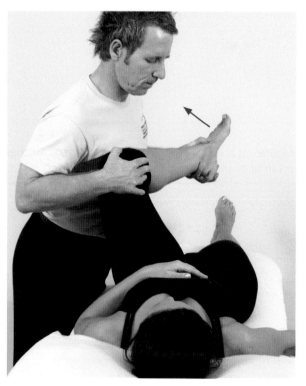

Figure 9.7 demonstrates my preferred way of lengthening the piriformis. Controlling the patient's left leg, the therapist tries to encourage flexion of the hip, while at the same time externally rotating the hip with some adduction. This technique will put the piriformis on a bind, but will need fine-tuning to get to the optimum position.

Note: It is known that after 60 degrees of hip flexion, the piriformis changes from an external rotator to an internal rotator – this is due to its anatomical attachments. If you look closely at the picture, this is the reason that the patient's left hip is placed in an externally rotated position. This will now lengthen the piriformis, as the left hip has greater than 60 degrees of flexion.

From the position of bind, the patient is asked to push their knee away, into the abdomen of the therapist. This will induce a contraction of the piriformis. After a 10-second contraction and on the relaxation phase, the therapist passively encourages the hip into further internal rotation while applying some hip adduction.

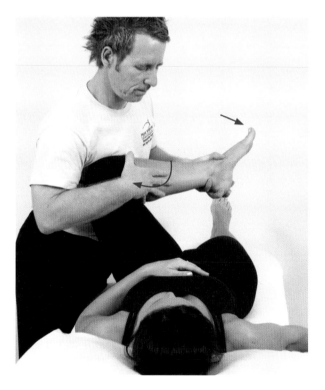

Figure 9.7: The therapist encourages further rotation of the left hip, using their chest and hand.

TIP: One in five of the population has the sciatic nerve passing through their piriformis muscle. This can result in buttock and leg pain, but generally no back pain is present, so make sure you eliminate disc pathology from your hypothesis.

Quadratus Lumborum

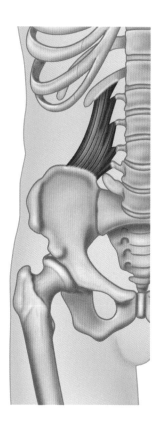

Origin

Iliac crest. Iliolumbar ligament (the ligament from the fifth lumbar vertebra to the ilium).

Insertion

Twelfth rib. Transverse processes of upper four lumbar vertebrae, (L1-L4).

Action

Laterally flexes vertebral column. Fixes the twelfth rib during deep respiration (e.g. helps stabilise the diaphragm of singers exercising voice control). Helps extend lumbar part of vertebral column and gives it lateral stability.

Nerve

Ventral rami of the subcostal nerve and upper three or four lumbar nerves (T12, L1, L2, L3).

Assessment of Quadratus Lumborum

In my experience I find that the standing side-flexion test is relatively good for indicating tightness of the QL.

The patient stands upright and maintains a neutral position of the lumbar spine. From the standing position, the patient is asked to side bend to the left, as shown in figure 9.8, and while side bending slides their left hand down the outside of their left leg. When the position of bind is reached (this is felt by the therapist palpating the right side of the QL as the patient side bends to the left), the patient's left middle finger should be in contact with the head of the fibula on the left side.

If the middle finger is close or touches the fibula head, the QL on the right (contralateral) side is classified as normal; if there is a restriction, the QL on the right is classified as tight.

Please note that this test is not conclusive for determining shortness of the QL, as many other lumbar spine factors will affect the overall result. For example, any discal or facet joint pain will be affected during this test and will give the therapist a false positive result.

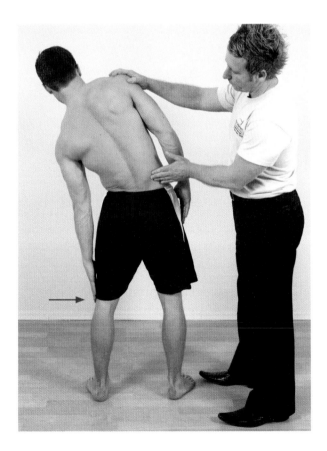

Figure 9.8: The left hand approximates the head of the fibula if the right QL is normal.

MET Treatment of Quadratus Lumborum

PIR Method

The patient is asked to adopt the shape of a 'banana'; this is achieved by the patient assuming a side-lying supine position, with their right hand placed underneath their head and their right leg over their left leg. The left leg overlays the edge of the couch, as shown in figure 9.9.

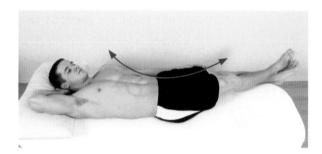

Figure 9.9: The QL is slightly at point of bind.

Once the patient has adopted this position, the therapist places their right hand under the head of the patient and cradles the right axilla. The left hand of the therapist stabilises the patient's left pelvis.

From this position, the patient is asked to side bend to the right against the resistance applied to their axilla by the therapist's right hand (figure 9.10). This will induce a contraction of their right QL.

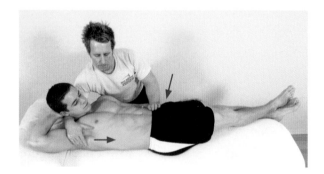

Figure 9.10: The patient side bends to the right while the therapist's left hand stabilises the patient's left pelvis.

After a 10-second contraction and on the relaxation phase, the therapist induces further side bending to the left, which will lengthen the QL on the right side.

RI Method

The position of the patient and the procedure is similar to that explained for the PIR method, the only difference being that when the therapist encourages the new position of bind, the patient is asked to reach their left hand towards their left leg (figure 9.11). This will induce a contraction of the left QL and cause the right QL to relax through RI, allowing a lengthening to occur.

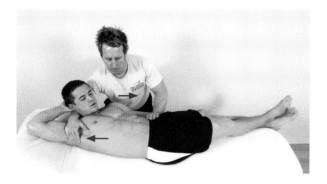

Figure 9.11: The therapist encourages side bending to the left.

Alternative METs for Quadratus Lumborum

For the first alternative MET, the patient is placed in a side-lying position, with their left leg off the side of the couch, as shown in figure 9.12. The therapist stabilises the lower back with their right hand and controls the patient's left leg with their left hand. The patient is asked to abduct their left leg against the resistance applied by the therapist's left hand; this will induce a contraction of the left QL.

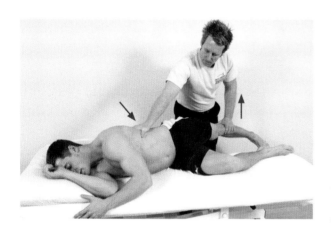

Figure 9.12: The patient abducts their left leg while the therapist's right hand stabilises the lower back.

After a 10-second contraction and on the relaxation phase, the therapist slowly and passively takes the patient's left leg into further adduction while stabilising the patient's lower back (figure 9.13). This will lengthen the QL on the left side.

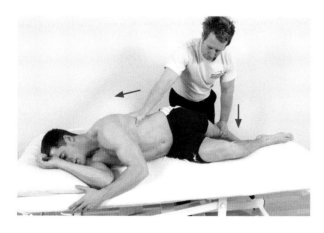

Figure 9.13: The therapist stabilises the lower back and gently applies cephalic pressure while encouraging adduction of the left leg.

The second alternative MET is performed with the patient in a side-lying position at the caudal end of the couch, with their left leg off the side of the couch, as shown in figure 9.14. The therapist steps over the patient's left leg and gently squeezes it with their thighs; the therapist also stabilises the patient's lower back with their right hand.

The patient is asked to abduct their left leg against the resistance applied by the therapist's thighs; this will induce a contraction of the left QL.

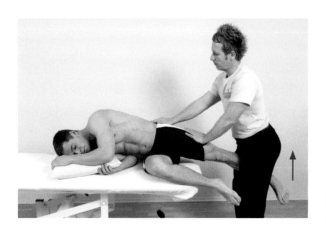

Figure 9.14: The patient abducts their leg against resistance applied by the therapist's thighs.

After a 10-second contraction and on the relaxation phase, the therapist slowly and passively takes the patient's left leg into further adduction by slowly squatting down, while at the same time cradling the patient's iliac crest. This will lengthen the QL on the left side.

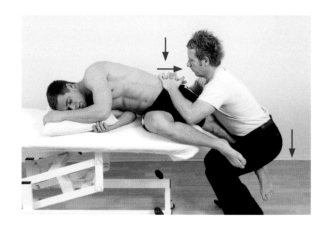

Figure 9.15: The therapist cradles the iliac crest and encourages caudal pressure while slowly bending down and lengthening the QL.

TIP: The QL can become overactive with subsequent shortening if the contralateral gluteus medius is weak.

Iliopsoas: Psoas Major and Iliacus

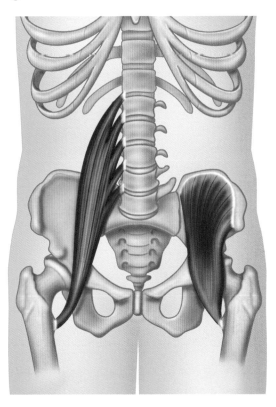

Origin

Psoas major: Transverse processes of all lumbar vertebrae (L1-L5). Bodies of twelfth thoracic and all lumbar vertebrae (T12-L5). Intervertebral discs above each lumbar vertebra.

Iliacus: Superior two-thirds of iliac fossa. Anterior ligaments of the lumbosacral and sacroiliac joints.

Insertion

Lesser trochanter of femur.

Action

Main flexor of hip joint and assists in lateral rotation of hip. Acting from its insertion, flexes the trunk, as in sitting up from the supine position.

Nerve

Psoas major: Ventral rami of lumbar nerves (L1, L2, L3, L4).

Iliacus: Femoral nerve (L1, L2, L3, L4).

Assessment of Iliopsoas

Modified Thomas Test
The patient is asked to lie back on the edge of a couch while holding onto their left knee. As they roll backwards, the patient pulls their left knee as far as they can towards their chest, as shown in figure 9.16. The full flexion of the hip encourages full posterior rotation of the pelvis and helps to flatten the lordosis.

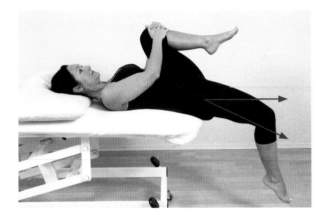

Figure 9.16: The knee is below the level of the hip, indicating a normal length of the psoas.

From this position, the therapist looks at where the patient's right knee lies, relative to the right hip. The position of the knee should be just below the level of the hip; figure 9.16 demonstrates a normal length of the right iliopsoas.

In figure 9.17 the therapist is demonstrating with their arms the position of the right hip compared to the right knee. You can see that the hip is held in a flexed position, which confirms the tightness of the right iliopsoas in this case.

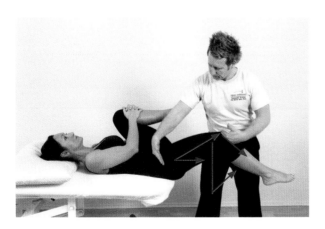

Figure 9.17: The knee is higher than the hip, indicating a tight right psoas. A tight rectus femoris is also seen here.

Note: In figure 9.17 you will also notice that the lower right leg is held in extension; this indicates a shortened right rectus femoris. (This was encountered in chapter 8).

Also from the position of the modified Thomas test, the therapist can apply an abduction of the hip, as demonstrated in figure 9.18, and an adduction of the hip, as demonstrated in figure 9.19. A range of motion of 10-15 degrees in both planes is commonly accepted to be normal from the modified Thomas position.

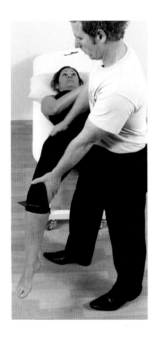   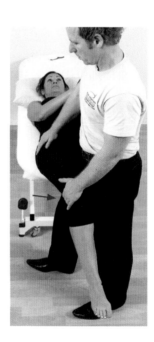

Figure 9.18: Abduction to indicate tight adductors.   *Figure 9.19: Adduction to indicate tight TFL/ITB.*

If the hip is restricted in abduction, i.e. a bind occurs at an angle less than 10-15 degrees, the muscles of the adductor group are held in a shortened position; if the adduction movement is restricted, the ITB and the TFL are held in a shortened position.

MET Treatment of Iliopsoas

The patient adopts the same position as for the test described earlier. After placing the patient's foot into their side, the therapist applies a pressure that induces full flexion of the patient's left hip. Stabilising the patient's right hip with their right hand, the therapist puts their left hand just above the patient's right knee. The patient is asked to flex their hip against a resistance for 10 seconds, as shown in figure 9.20.

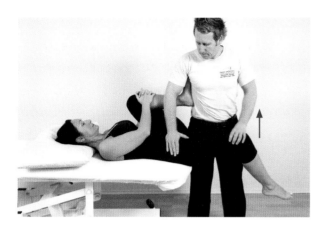

Figure 9.20: The patient flexes their right hip against the therapist's resistance. The therapist is stabilising the right hip with their right hand.

After the isometric contraction and on the relaxation phase, the therapist slowly applies a downward pressure. This will cause the hip to passively go into extension and will cause a lengthening of the right psoas, as shown in figure 9.21. Gravity will also play a part in this technique, as it will assist the lengthening of the psoas.

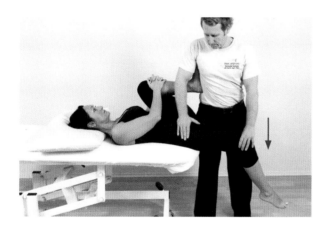

Figure 9.21: The therapist passively extends the hip to lengthen the psoas, assisted by gravity.

An alternative way of contracting the iliopsoas is possible from the flexed position shown in figure 9.22. This is normally used if the original way of activating the iliopsoas causes discomfort to the patient. Allowing the hip to be in a more flexed position will slacken the iliopsoas – this will assist in its contraction and help reduce the discomfort.

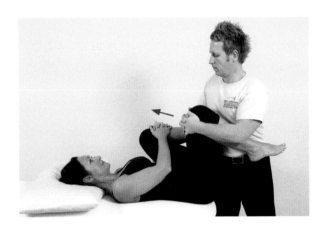

Figure 9.22: From the flexed position, the patient is asked to resist hip flexion.

The patient is asked to flex their hip against a resistance applied by the therapist's left hand, as shown in figure 9.22. After a 10-second contraction and on the relaxation phase, the therapist lengthens the iliopsoas by taking the hip into an extended position, as demonstrated in figure 9.23.

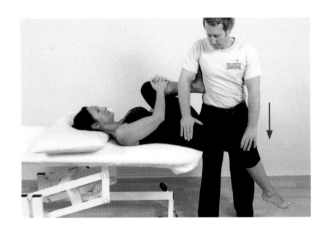

Figure 9.23: Lengthening of the right psoas.

TIP: The psoas major is also known as filet mignon, which is a piece of beef taken from the tenderloin. A bilateral shortness of the psoas can cause the pelvis to anteriorly tilt and cause the lumbar spine to adopt a position of hyperlordosis. This can cause compression of the facet joints and the patient will present with lower back pain.

Note: If full sit-ups are performed on a regular basis, the psoas muscle is predominantly being used. Repeated sit-ups will make the psoas stronger and tighter, and result in weakness of the abdominals; this can maintain a patient's lower back pain.

To prove the involvement of the psoas, have your patient lie on their back with their knees bent. Hold the patient's ankles and ask them to dorsiflex their ankles while you resist the movement. This will stimulate the anterior chain musculature, including the psoas, which is part of this chain. The patient then performs the sit-up movement (most fit individuals will be able to do many sit-ups).

To deactivate or switch off the psoas, we ask the patient to plantar flex their ankles (instead of dorsiflexing them), or to squeeze their gluteals. Either of these actions stimulates the posterior chain musculature, causing the psoas to switch off, as activation of the gluteal muscles results in a relaxation of the psoas through reciprocal inhibition. When the patient is now asked to perform the sit-up, the movement will prove to be impossible, confirming that the psoas is generally the prime mover in a full sit-up.

Erector Spinae

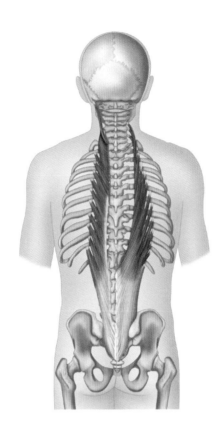

Origin
Slips of muscle arising from the sacrum. Iliac crest. Spinous and transverse processes of vertebrae. Ribs.

Insertion
Ribs. Transverse and spinous processes of vertebrae. Occipital bone.

Action
Extends and laterally flexes vertebral column (i.e. bending backwards and sideways). Helps maintain correct curvature of spine in the erect and sitting positions. Steadies the vertebral column on the pelvis during walking.

Nerve
Dorsal rami of cervical, thoracic and lumbar spinal nerves.

Assessment of Erector Spinae

Figures 9.24-9.27 demonstrate a test for identifying tightness in the erector spinae muscles, using the same position as for a sit and reach test. Note that this test will identify if there is tightness in the hamstrings, gastrocnemius and soleus, as well as in the erector spinae muscles.

The test is done with the patient in a long sitting position with their knees bent. The patient is asked to bend forwards, with their hands outstretched in an attempt to touch their toes, as shown in figure 9.24. If this can be achieved, and at the same time the ankle is able to dorsiflex to 90 degrees, there is probably normal length of all the muscles of the lower back, hamstrings, gastrocnemius and soleus.

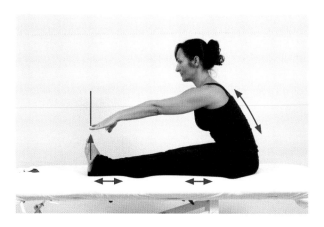

Figure 9.24: The patient is demonstrating normal length of all the muscles of the lower back, hamstrings, gastrocnemius and soleus.

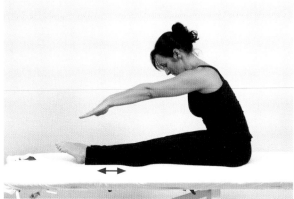

Figure 9.25: The patient is able to reach their toes with their fingers, but their ankle is plantar flexing (pointing downwards), which indicates tightness in their gastrocnemius and soleus.

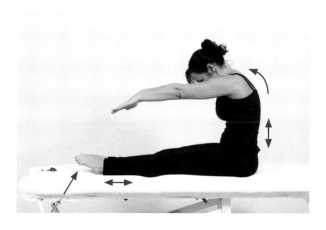

Figure 9.26: The patient is unable to touch their toes, and their lower back does not seem to flex to a natural curved position, so one can assume that the muscles of the erector spinae are held in a shortened position. Also, note that the ankle is plantar flexed, indicating tightness of the gastrocnemius and soleus.

Figure 9.27(a) demonstrates the patient's inability to touch their toes, even though their lower back is slightly rounded. The patient will be feeling tension in the back of the posterior part of the upper leg; this indicates that the hamstrings are held in a shortened position. Hamstring shortness will hold the pelvis in a posteriorly rotated position, and when this occurs the lumbar spine will only be capable of a small amount of flexion. This will compromise and load the intervertebral disc, which can then lead to pain.

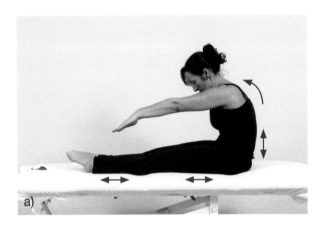 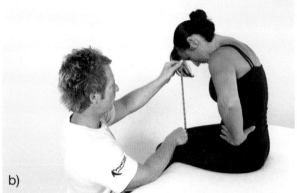

Figure 9.27: (a) Tight lower back muscles, hamstrings and gastrocnemius; (b) Measurement is taken from the forehead to the thigh, before the treatment.

You will also notice in figure 9.27(a) that the ankles are held in plantar flexion, indicating tightness of the gastrocnemius and soleus.

Specific test for the length of the lumbar spine erector

The patient sits on the end of a couch and is asked to roll their chin down to their chest, and to continue flexing down, vertebra by vertebra. The therapist palpates the top of the patient's iliac crest and the PSIS with their thumbs, and when they feel the muscular tension increase to their hands, the test is complete. A measurement of more than 15 cm, or 8 inches, from the patient's forehead to the top of their knees indicates a tight lumbar erector spinae (figure 9.27(b)).

MET Treatment of Lumbar Spine Erector Spinae

The patient adopts a prone position with a pillow placed under their abdomen. The therapist places their left hand on the patient's lower thoracic spine and their right hand on the patient's sacrum, as shown in figure 9.28(a). The patient is asked to lift their shoulders off the couch to contract the lumbar erector spinae (figure 9.28(a)).

After a 10-second contraction and on the relaxation phase, the therapist takes their left hand into a more cephalic position and their right hand into a more caudal position. This separation of the therapist's hands will encourage the lengthening of the lumbar spine erector spinae (figure 9.28(b)). Once an MET has been performed for the erector spinae, the therapist can reassess the length of these muscles, to see if there is an improvement, as shown in figure 9.28(c).

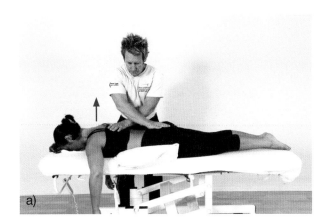

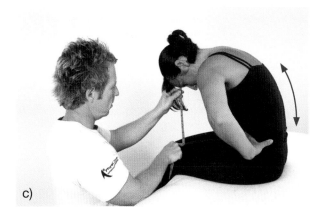

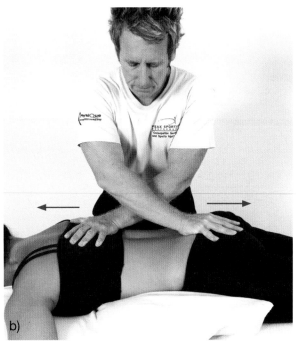

Figure 9.28: MET treatment of lumbar spine erector spinae. (a) Hand position demonstrated by the therapist as the patient lifts their shoulder blades to contract the muscles; (b) The therapist separates their hands to encourage lengthening of the patient's erector spinae; (c) A measurement is taken again after the MET treatment; further length is achieved of the erector spinae after treatment.

TIP: In a lower crossed syndrome (where the patient has an anterior tilt of the pelvis), the lumbar spine erector spinae will normally be held in a shortened position. The consequence of this muscular shortness is that the lumbar spine will be encouraged to increase its lordosis and cause lower back pain.

Specific Testing for Muscle Weakness

10

There are lots of books on muscle testing, but I would like to cover some of the muscles that can become weakened as a result of specific tightness. However, when I say a muscle is weak, this might not be true for certain muscles. For example, part of this chapter will look at the firing pattern movement of hip extension and we specifically look for a 'mis' firing sequence, i.e. the muscle is slower to contract. This does not necessarily mean the muscle is weak – it can simply mean it is firing to contract in the wrong order. If I tested the strength of the gluteus maximus, for instance, that is showing to be misfiring (i.e. contracting in an incorrect sequence), I may assume this muscle is weak. However, if I were to isololate and specifically test the gluteus maximus for strength, it would probably test as normal (graded scale of 5, see table 10.1).

Grade	Description
0	No muscle movement
1	Visible muscle movement, but no movement at the joint
2	Movement at the joint, but not against gravity
3	Movement against gravity, but not against added resistance
4	Movement against resistance, but less than normal
5	Normal strength

Table 10.1: Muscle grades of motor strength.

If you remember, in previous chapters, I talked about two main types of muscle – postural and phasic. I have described the majority of the postural muscles, as these are prone to shortening and tightening. In this chapter we are going to look at the phasic muscles: these muscles of power are prone to lengthening and weakening.

Janda (1983) demonstrated that lengthening the shortened tight tissues of the erector spinae caused the apparently lengthened and weakened rectus abdominus to contract more effectively. His study proves that it is more appropriate to 'lengthen before you strengthen'. If you follow this simple analogy, it could work very well with your patients in your own clinic.

This chapter will look at certain muscles that might have become lengthened and then weakened as a result of the antagonistic muscles becoming adaptively shortened. Sherrington's law of reciprocal inhibition confirms part of this process and explains what may be responsible for causing this and holding the phasic muscles in a lengthened position.

The following muscles will be tested and treated for weakness:

- Gluteus maximus (Gmax)
- Gluteus medius (Gmed)
- Serratus anterior
- Lower fibres of the trapezius

MUSCLE WEAKNESS ASSESSMENT SHEET

Patient Name:

Key: E = Equal

L/R = Weak on left or right side

Muscles	Date:	Date:	Date:
Gluteus maximus			
Gluteus medius			
Posterior fibres of gluteus medius			
Serratus anterior			
Lower fibres of trapezius			

Gluteus Maximus (Gmax)

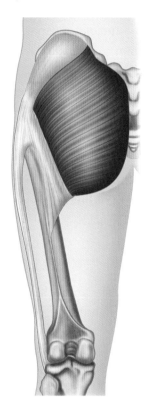

Origin

Outer surface of ilium behind posterior gluteal line and portion of bone superior and posterior to it. Adjacent posterior surface of sacrum and coccyx. Sacrotuberous ligament. Aponeurosis of erector spinae.

Insertion

Deep fibres of distal portion: gluteal tuberosity of femur.
Remaining fibres: iliotibial tract of fascia lata.

Action

Upper fibres: laterally rotate hip joint. May assist in abduction of hip joint.
Lower fibres: extend and laterally rotate hip joint (forceful extension as in running or rising from sitting). Extend trunk. Assists in adduction of hip joint.
Through its insertion into the iliotibial tract, helps to stabilize the knee in extension.

Nerve

Inferior gluteal nerve, L5, S1, 2.

Function of Gluteus Maximus

From a functional perspective, the Gmax performs several key roles in controlling the relationship between the pelvis, trunk and femur. This muscle is capable of abducting and laterally rotating the hip, which helps to control the alignment of the knee with the lower limb. For example, in stair climbing, the Gmax will laterally rotate and abduct the hip to keep the lower limb in optimal alignment, while at the same time the hip extends to carry the body upwards onto the next step. When the Gmax is weak or misfiring, the knee can be seen to deviate medially and the pelvis can also be observed to tip laterally.

The Gmax also has a role in stabilising the sacroiliac joints (SIJs) and has been described as one of the force closure muscles. Some of the Gmax fibres attach to the sacrotuberous ligament and the thoracolumbar fascia, which is a very strong, non-contractile connective tissue that is tensioned by the activation of muscles connecting to it. One of the connections to this fascia is the latissimus dorsi. The Gmax forms a partnership with the contralateral latissimus dorsi via the thoracolumbar fascia – this partnership connection is known as the posterior oblique sling. This sling increases the compression force to the sacroiliac joint during the weight-bearing single-leg stance in the gait cycle.

Posterior Oblique Sling

The posterior oblique sling consists of:

Gluteus maximus
Contralateral latissimus dorsi
Thoracolumbar fascia.

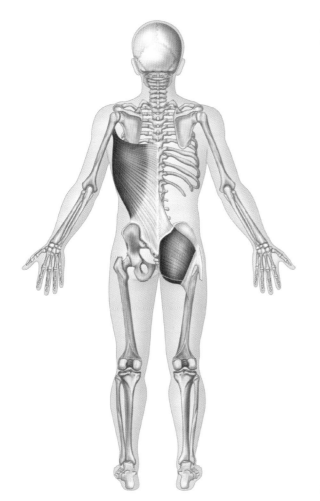

Figure 10.1: Posterior oblique sling.

Misfiring or weakness in the Gmax reduces the effectiveness of the posterior oblique sling, which will predispose the SIJs to subsequent injury. The body will then try to compensate for this weakness by increasing tension via the thoracolumbar fascia by in turn increasing the activation of the contralateral latissimus dorsi. As with any compensatory mechanism, 'structure affects function' and 'function affects structure'. This means that other areas of the body are affected: the shoulder mechanics are altered due to the attachment of the latissimus dorsi on the humerus and scapula. If the latissimus dorsi is particularly active due to the compensation, this can be seen as one shoulder appears lower than the other during a step-up or even a lunge type of motion.

The Gmax plays a significant role in the gait cycle, working in conjunction with the hamstrings. Just before heel strike, the hamstrings will activate, which will increase the tension to the SIJs via the attachment on the sacrotuberous ligament. This connection assists in the locking mechanism of the SIJs for the weight-bearing cycle. From heel strike to mid-stance of the gait, the Gmax increases its activation and the hamstrings decrease their activation. The Gmax significantly increases the stabilisation of the SIJs during early and mid-stance phases through the attachments of the posterior oblique sling.

Weakness or misfiring in the Gmax will cause the hamstrings to remain active during the gait cycle, to maintain stability of the SIJs and the position of the pelvis. The resultant overactivation of the hamstrings during the gait cycle will subject them to continual and abnormal strain.

Hip Extension Firing Pattern Test

Figure 10.2 indicates the correct firing pattern of hip joint extension. The normal muscle activation sequence is:

1. Gluteus maximus
2. Hamstrings
3. Contralateral lumbar extensors
4. Ipsilateral lumbar extensors
5. Contralateral thoracolumbar extensors
6. Ipsilateral thoracolumbar extensors

Note that ideally the gluteus maximus activates first, followed by the hamstrings, although it is acceptable if the two fire simultaneously.

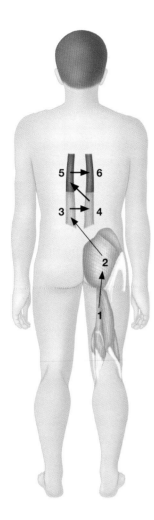

Muscle activation sequence

1. Hamstrings
2. Gluteus maximus
3. Contralateral lumbar extensors
4. Ipsilateral lumbar extensors
5. Contralateral thoracolumbar extensors
6. Ipsilateral thoracolumbar extensors

Either group may normally activate first

Figure 10.2: Correct firing pattern of hip joint extension.

The hip extension firing pattern test is very unique in its application. Think of yourself as a six-cylinder engine: basically that is what our body is – an engine. The engine has a certain way of firing and so does our body. For example, the engine in a car will not fire its individual cylinders in the order 1–2–3–4–5–6; it will fire in the sequence, say, 1–3–5–6–4–2.

If we have our car serviced and the mechanic mistakes two of the leads and puts them back incorrectly, the engine will still work but will not be very efficient; over time, the engine will start to break down. Our body is no different: in our case, if we are particularly active but have a misfiring dysfunction, our body will also break down and eventually cause us to experience pain.

Sequence 1

The therapist places their fingertips lightly on the patient's left hamstrings and left gluteus maximus (figure 10.3(a) and (b)), and the patient is asked to lift their left leg two inches off the couch (figure 10.4). The therapist tries to identify which muscle fires first and notes the first sequence.

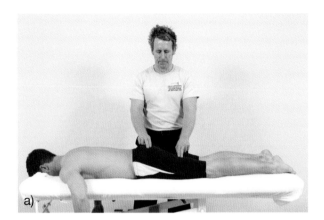

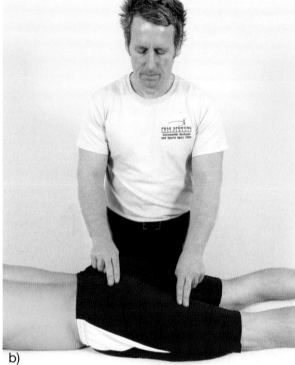

Figure 10.3: Sequence 1. (a) The therapist lightly palpates the patient's left hamstrings and Gmax; (b) Close-up view of the therapist's hand position.

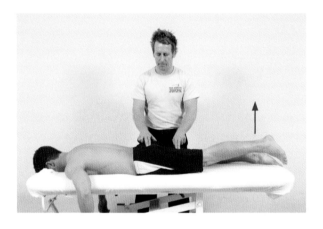

Figure 10.4: Sequence 1. The patient lifts their left leg off the couch.

Sequence 2

The therapist places their thumbs lightly on the patient's erector spinae, and the patient is asked to lift their left leg two inches off the couch (figures 10.5 and 10.6). The therapist identifies and notes which erector muscle fires first.

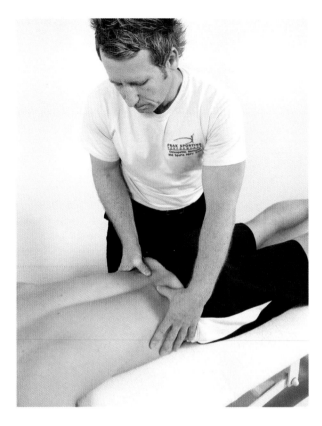

Figure 10.5: Sequence 2. The therapist lightly palpates the patient's erector spinae.

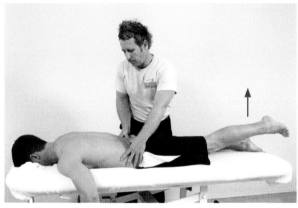

Figure 10.6: Sequence 2. The patient lifts their left leg off the couch.

Once the results of sequences 1 and 2 have been recorded (see tables 10.2 and 10.3), the therapist then has to decide what order the muscles fire in. The normal sequence will be: (1) gluteus maximus, (2) hamstrings, (3) contralateral erector and, lastly, (4) ipsilateral erector spinae. So this will be the correct firing pattern.

If, when palpating in sequence 1, the gluteus maximus is found to fire first, you can safely say that this is correct. The same applies in sequence 2: if the contralateral erector spinae contracts first, this is also the correct sequence.

However, if you feel that the hamstrings are number 1 in the sequence, or that the ipsilateral erector spinae is number 1 in the sequence and the gluteus maximus is not felt to contract, you can deduce that this is a misfiring pattern. If the misfiring dysfunction is not corrected, the engine (our body) will start to break down and a compensatory pattern of dysfunction will be formed.

	1st	2nd	3rd	4th
Gluteus maximus	○	○	○	○
Hamstrings	○	○	○	○
Contralateral erector spinae	○	○	○	○
Ipsilateral erector spinae	○	○	○	○

Table 10.2: Hip extension firing pattern – left side.

	1st	2nd	3rd	4th
Gluteus maximus	○	○	○	○
Hamstrings	○	○	○	○
Contralateral erector spinae	○	○	○	○
Ipsilateral erector spinae	○	○	○	○

Table 10.3: Hip extension firing pattern – right side.

In my experience I find that the hamstrings and the ipsilateral erector spinae are generally first to contract and the gluteus maximus is number four in the sequence. This will mean that the erector spinae and the hamstrings will become the dominant muscles in assisting the hip in an extension movement. This can cause excessive anterior tilting of the pelvis with a resultant hyperlordosis, which can lead to the lower lumbar facet joints becoming inflamed.

To correct the misfiring sequence, we need to look at the previous chapters on muscle length testing and the use of METs to treat shortened and tight tissues. The focus of this book has been to identify soft-tissue structures that are prone to shortening and becoming tight. I have already discussed 'why' the antagonistic muscles can become lengthened and weakened; this is applicable to the Gmax and, later on in this chapter, the gluteus medius (Gmed), as they are both part of the phasic muscle group. The answer is not to strengthen the so-called 'weak' muscles, since encouraging strength-based exercise will not assist these specific muscles in regaining their muscular strength.

Remember which muscles are antagonistic to the Gmax? Well, the Gmax is a powerful hip extensor so it has to be the hip flexors – the main muscles responsible for hip flexion are the psoas, rectus femoris and adductors. One way of encouraging a correct firing pattern is to identify the length of the hip flexors: if they are tested as short, an MET can be utilised to assist in normalising the resting length of these shortened structures. This theory of lengthening the shortened structures can be applied for a period of approximately two weeks; if the firing pattern has not improved in this two-week period, strengthening protocols for the Gmax can then be incorporated into the treatment plan.

Note: The firing patterns of muscles 5 and 6 have not been discussed in this chapter, because we need to make sure that the correct firing order of muscles 1–4 is established. I also find that when the muscle 1–4 firing sequence has been corrected, the firing pattern of muscles 5 and 6 is generally self-correcting and tends to follow the normal firing pattern sequence.

Athlete presents with	What can it imply?	Likely finding
Tight/painful hamstrings or lumbar paraspinal muscles	Faulty posterior chain muscle activation pattern	GMax weakness or delayed timing on same side
Insufficient forward or upward power production from the legs		
Pelvic position dropped when running		
Tight/painful adductor magnus (inner thigh) Asymmetrical body orientation	Faulty hip extension pattern: adductor magnus being over used to extend the hip	GMax function decreased on same side
Asymmetrical body orientation		
Better balance one side than the other		
Excessively tight latissimus dorsi (remembering that the dominant arm will often be slightly less flexible than the non-dominant one)	Faulty posterior oblique sling	GMax function decreased on opposite side

Table 10.4: GMax summary. Taken from: 'Sport, Stability and Performance Movement: great technique without injury: Elphinston, J., Lotus Publishing, 2008.

Gluteus Medius (Gmed)

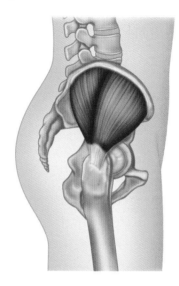

Origin

Outer surface of ilium inferior to iliac crest, between the posterior gluteal line and the anterior gluteal line.

Insertion

Oblique ridge on lateral surface of greater trochanter of femur.

Action

Upper fibres: laterally rotate hip joint. May assist in abduction of hip joint.

Abducts the hip joint. Anterior fibres medially rotate and may assist in flexion of the hip joint. Posterior fibres slightly laterally rotate the hip joint.

Nerve

Superior gluteal nerve, L4, 5, S1.

Assessment of Gluteus Medius

'A strong Gmax and Gmed is a stable knee'

Whenever I look at patients who present with knee or lower lumbar spine pain, part of my assessment process includes checking the strength of the gluteal muscles. We discussed the hip extension firing order earlier in this chapter to determine the correct firing order; now we are going to look at the function of the gluteus medius (Gmed) and then how to test the Gmed functionally.

Function of Gluteus Medius

The Gmed is predominantly used in the gait cycle, especially during the initial contact with the ground and the stance phase of the cycle. Broadly speaking, the Gmed is responsible for maintaining the position of the pelvis as we walk from A to B.

The Gmed has a posterior fibre in its structure as well as an anterior component; it is the posterior fibres that we as therapists are concerned with. The Gmed posterior fibres work in conjunction with the Gmax, and these muscles control the position of the hip into an external rotation, which helps to align the hip, knee and lower limb as the gait cycle is initiated.

As an example, consider a patient who is asked to walk while the therapist observes the process. As the patient's weight is applied to their left leg at the initial contact phase of the cycle, the Gmed is responsible for part of the stability mechanism acting on the lower limb; this will also assist in the overall alignment of the lower limb. The patient continues with the gait cycle and is now in the stance phase. The Gmed in this phase is responsible for abducting the right hip; the right hip is then seen to start to lift slightly higher than the left side. This process is very important as it allows the right leg to swing during the swing phase of gait.

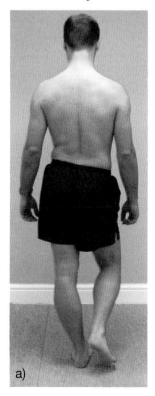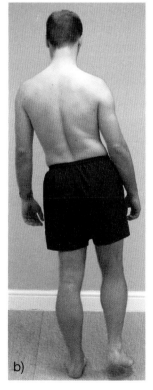

a)   b)

Figure 10.7: a) Trendelenburg gait; b) compensatory Trendelenburg gait. Taken from: 'Sport, Stability and Performance Movement: great technique without injury: Elphinston, J., Lotus Publishing, 2008.

If there is any weakness in the left Gmed, the body will respond in two ways during the gait cycle: either the pelvis will tip down on the contralateral side to the stance leg (right in this case), giving the appearance of a 'Trendelenburg' pattern of gait (figure10.7a); or a 'compensatory Trendelenburg' pattern will be adopted, in which the patient is observed to shift their whole trunk excessively to the weaker hip (figure 10.7b).

When we stand on one leg, we activate the lateral sling, which consists of the gluteus medius, gluteus minimus, adductors on the ipsilateral side, and the quadratus lumborum on the contralateral side. As explained earlier, if we present with weakness, this is probably a result of overactivation in other muscles due to the compensation process. Patients who present with weakness in their Gmed (posterior fibres) tend to have overactivity of the adductors and iliotibial band via the connection from the tensor fasciae latae; also the piriformis has an overactive role if the Gmed posterior fibres are shown to be weak.

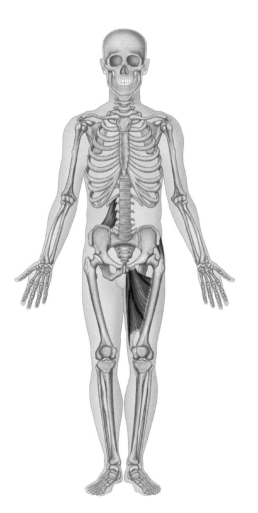

Lateral Sling
The lateral sling consists of:

Gluteus medius and minimus
(abductors of the hip)
Ipsilateral (same side) adductors
of the hip
Contralateral (opposite side) quadratus
lumborum

Figure 10.8: Lateral sling.

We are now going to look at the 'firing order' of a hip abduction movement, to decide if the Gmed is firing normally.

Hip Abduction Firing Pattern Test

The patient adopts a side-lying posture with both legs together. In this sequence, three muscles will be tested: gluteus medius (Gmed), tensor fasciae latae (TFL) and quadratus lumborum (QL). The QL muscle is palpated by the therapist placing their right hand lightly on the muscle (figure 10.9). Next, the Gmed and TFL are palpated by the therapist placing their finger on the TFL and their thumb on the Gmed.

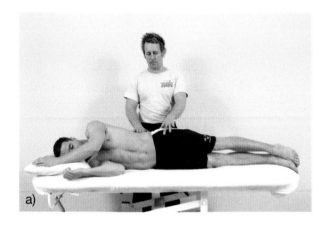

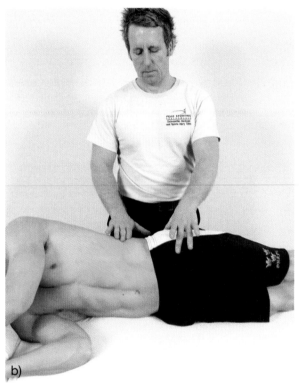

Figure 10.9: (a) Palpation of the QL, Gmed, and TFL; (b) Close-up of the hand position.

The patient is asked to lift their left leg into abduction a few inches from their right leg, and the therapist notes the firing sequence (figure 10.10).

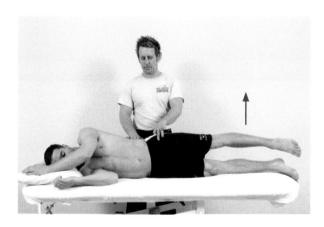

Figure 10.10: The therapist notes the firing sequence as the patient abducts their left leg.

The correct firing sequence should be gluteus medius, followed by TFL, and finally QL at around 25 degrees of pelvis elevation. If the QL or the TFL were to fire first, this would indicate a misfiring sequence, resulting in adaptive shortness.

Once we have ascertained the firing sequence for the hip abduction firing pattern, we have to decide on the next step. Most patients feel that they need to strengthen the weak Gmed muscle by going to the gym, especially if they have been told it is weak, and they do lots of side-lying abduction exercises. The difficulty in strengthening the apparent weak Gmed muscle is that this particular exercise will not, I repeat will not, strengthen the Gmed, especially if the TFL and QL are the dominant abductors. The piriformis will also get involved as it is a weak abductor, which can cause a pelvic/sacroiliac dysfunction, further complicating the underlying issue.

So the answer to the question is to leave the strengthening of the Gmed initially and focus on the shortened/tight tissues of the adductors, TFL and QL. In theory, by lengthening the tight tissues, the lengthened and weakened tissue then becomes shorter and can automatically regain its strength. If, after a period of time (two weeks has been recommended) the Gmed has not regained its strength, specific and functional strength exercises for this muscle can be added.

Gluteus Medius Anterior/Posterior Fibres Strength Test

The patient adopts a side-lying posture. The therapist palpates the patient's Gmed with their right hand, and the patient is asked to abduct their left hip a few inches off the right leg. The patient holds this position isometrically to start with. The therapist then places their left hand near the patient's knee and applies a downward pressure to the leg, and the patient is asked to resist the pressure (figure 10.11). If the patient is able to resist the pressure that is being applied, the Gmed is classified as normal.

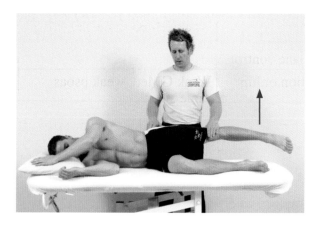

Figure 10.11: The patient abducts their left hip against resistance from the therapist.

Gluteus Medius Posterior Fibres Strength Test

In figure 10.12, the therapist is controlling the patient's left leg into slight extension and external rotation, to put more emphasis on the posterior fibres of the Gmed. As before, the therapist applies a downward pressure (figure 10.13), and if the patient is able to resist this force, the Gmed posterior fibres are classified as normal.

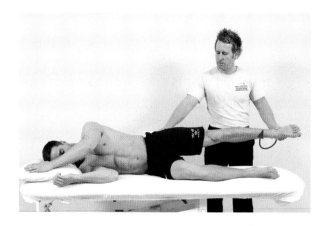

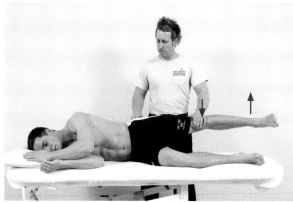

Figure 10.12: External rotation of the hip emphasises the posterior fibres of the Gmed.

Figure 10.13: The therapist applies downward pressure to the abducted hip of the patient.

Athlete presents with	What can it imply?	Likely finding
Swagger or pendulum gait	Faulty weight bearing strategy	Weak GMed
Tight quadratus lumborum (side trunk muscles)	Difficulty orientating the trunk vertically over the pelvis in gait, requiring overuse of side trunk muscles	Weak GMed opposite side
Tight piriformis	Faulty pelvic control in weight bearing requiring greater coronal plane control	Weak GMed same side
Tight ITB/lateral knee pain/ knee cap pain	Faulty hip abduction or hip flexion strategy	Weak GMed, weak psoas same side

Table 10.5: GMed summary. Taken from: 'Sport, Stability and Performance Movement: great technique without injury: Elphinston, J., Lotus Publishing, 2008.

Serratus Anterior

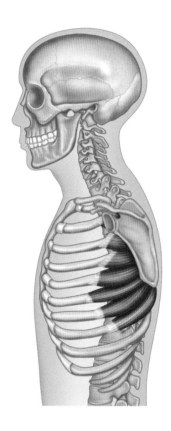

Origin

Outer surfaces and superior borders of upper eight or nine ribs, and the fascia covering their intercostal spaces.

Insertion

Anterior (costal) surface of the medial border of scapula and inferior angle of scapula.

Action

Rotates scapula for abduction and flexion of arm. Protracts scapula (pulls it forward on the chest wall and holds it closely in to the chest wall), facilitating pushing movements such as press-ups or punching.

Nerve

Long thoracic nerve, C5, 6, 7, 8.

Assessment of Serratus Anterior

Wall Push-Up Test

The wall push-up test is a low-load movement, which looks at coordination of the shoulder girdle with the trunk. For this test, we are specifically looking at the position of the scapula as it rotates around the rib cage. Another variation of the test is where the therapist observes the positions of the trunk, head and abdomen of the patient, with obvious deviations from the normal indicating that other dysfunctions are present. However, those dysfunctions will not be addressed in this book.

In a standing position, the patient places their hands on a wall at shoulder height in front of them, with their arms straight, as shown in figure 10.14. They are asked to bend their elbows to perform a 'push-up' movement against the wall.

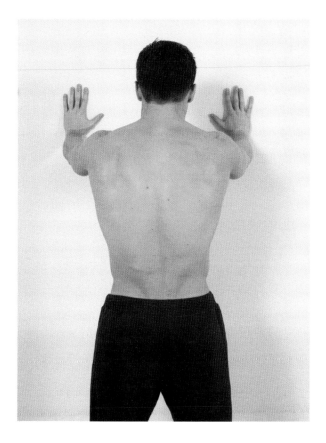

Figure 10.14: Starting position – the normal position of the scapula.

From this position, the patient performs the push-up and eccentrically controls the movement against the wall by the use of their pectorals, as demonstrated in figure 10.15. The therapist observes the motion of the scapula as the patient performs this movement.

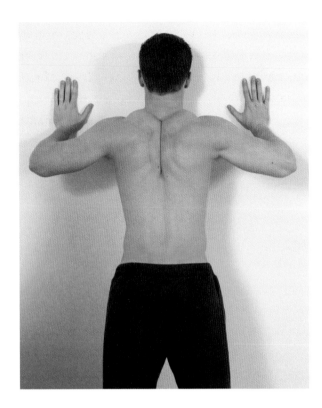

Figure 10.15: Part 1 – the normal retracted scapula position.

Figure 10.16 shows a normal scapula position and is indicated by the position of the scapula against the rib cage, with no signs of 'winging' of the scapula. This confirms a normal grading of the serratus anterior.

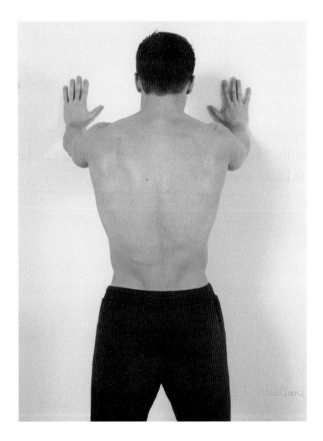

Figure 10.16: Part 2 – the normal position of the scapula against the rib cage.

Figure 10.17(a) shows a 'winging' of the right scapula, which might indicate a weakness of the right serratus anterior or possibly damage to the nerve that supplies the serratus anterior. This nerve is known as the long thoracic nerve and originates at the cervical spine level of C5, C6 and C7. A patient having a previous history of shoulder dislocations that have caused long-term damage to the long thoracic nerve may exhibit excessive 'winging' of the scapula (figure 10.17(b)).

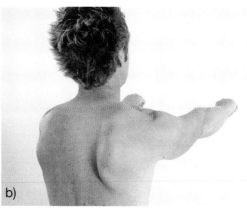

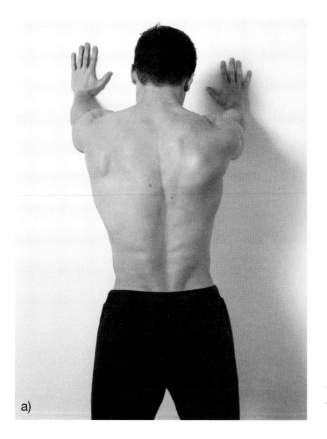

Figure 10.17: (a) Winging of the right scapula, indicating loss of scapula control; (b) Excessive winging of the right scapula.

Scapula Protraction Test

An alternative to the standing wall push-up test is the 'scapula protraction test', which can be done with the patient supine, as shown in figure 10.18, or seated, as in figure 10.19.

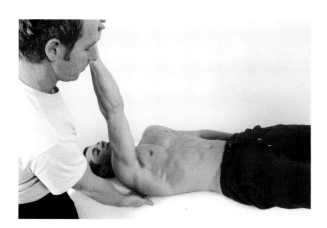

Figure 10.18: Patient lying supine as the therapist palpates the medial border of the right scapula while applying pressure to the patient's right fist.

The patient is asked to place their arm to 90 degrees of flexion with their hand clenched; the therapist grips the patient's clenched hand and palpates the medial border of the patient's right scapula. The therapist applies a pressure to the patient's clenched fist and tries to force the scapula into a 'retracted' position while the patient resists the pressure. If the scapula is felt to 'wing', a weakness of the serratus anterior is noted.

Figure 10.19(a) shows a normal scapula position without any 'winging'. However, you will note in figure 10.19(b) that this patient has excessive 'winging' of their right scapula – this is demonstrated even without pressure being applied by the therapist.

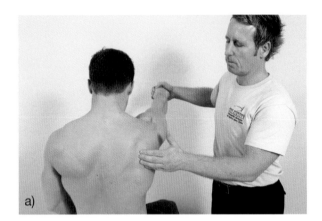 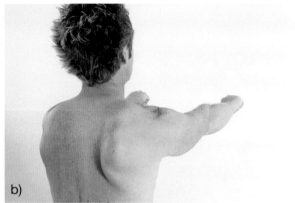

Figure 10.19: The therapist palpates for 'winging' of the right scapula. (a) A normal scapula position without any 'winging'; (b) The patient demonstrates excessive 'winging'.

Lower Fibres of Trapezius

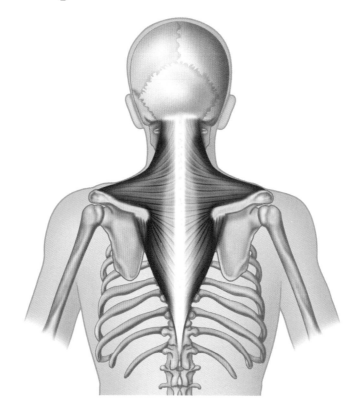

Origin

Medial third of superior nuchal line of occipital bone. External occipital protuberance. Ligamentum nuchae. Spinous processes and supraspinous ligaments of seventh cervical vertebra, (C7) and all thoracic vertebrae, (T1–T12).

Insertion

Medial border of crest of the spine of scapula, and the tubercle on this crest.

Action

Depresses scapula, particularly against resistance, as when using the hands to get up from a chair, and with the upper fibres, rotates scapula, as in elevating the arm above the head.

Nerve

Motor supply: Accessory X1 nerve.
Sensory supply (proprioception): Ventral ramus of cervical nerves, C2, 3, 4.

Assessment of Lower Fibres of Trapezius
Prone Arm Retraction Test

The patient adopts a prone position on the couch (figure 10.19), or they can be tested in a seated position (figure 10.20).

The patient is asked to place their arm at approximately 140 degrees of abduction, as shown in the figure. The therapist applies a downward pressure to the patient's left arm and palpates the patient's lower trapezius with their left hand.

The patient is asked to resist the pressure applied by the therapist; if the patient is able to resist the pressure, a normal grade of the lower trapezius is noted. The therapist notes if the patient is unable to resist the pressure, or if the scapula is seen to 'wing' slightly from the rib cage.

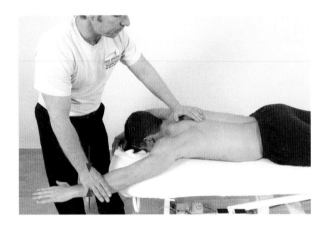

Figure 10.20: The patient (prone) resists the pressure applied by the therapist.

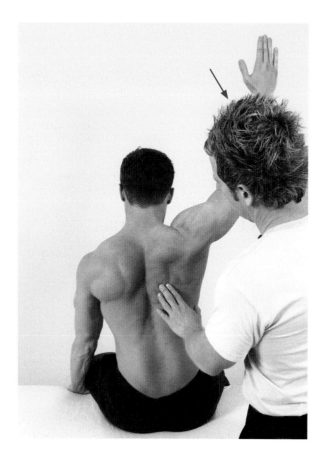

Figure 10.21: The patient (seated) resists the pressure applied by the therapist.

The therapist asks the patient to resist the pressure applied to their right arm and palpates the patient's right lower trapezius at the same time.

Weakness of the lower trapezius is a common occurrence in athletes; one reason for this, in my opinion, is that the afflicted athletes are 'pec dominant'. This implies that their pectorals are overactive and have developed into a shortened and tight state. To assist in regaining strength of the weakened lower trapezius, a relative shortness in the pectoralis minor and major must have been identified (see Chapter 7). Once the shortened pectorals have been identified as being tight, a lengthening programme using the MET techniques described in this book can be initiated. If, after a period of approximately two weeks, a weakness in the lower trapezius persists, a strengthening protocol can then be incorporated.

References

Abernethy, B., Hanrahan, S., Kippers, V., MacKinnon, T., & Pandy, M.: 2004. *The Biophysical Foundations of Human Movement*. Human Kinetics, Champaign, USA.

Caillet, R.: 2003. *The Illustrated Guide to Functional Anatomy of the Musculoskeletal System*. The American Medical Association, USA.

Chaitow, L.: 2006. *Muscle Energy Techniques, Second Edition*. Churchill Livingstone, Edinburgh.

Chek, P.: 2009. *An Integrated Approach to Stretching*. C.H.E.K. Institute. CA, USA.

Earls, J. & Myers, T.: *Fascial Release for Structural Balance*. Lotus Publishing, Chichester, UK/North Atlantic Books, Berkeley, USA.

Elphinston, J.: 2008. *Stability, Sport and Performance Movement: Great Technique Without Injury*. Lotus Publishing, Chichester, UK/North Atlantic Books, Berkeley, USA.

Hammer, W.: 1999. *Functional Soft Tissue Examination and Treatment by Manual Methods, New Perspectives, Second Edition*. Aspen, New York, USA.

Janda, V.: 1983. *Muscle Function Testing*. Butterworth-Heinemann, London, UK.

Jarmey, C.: 2008. *The Concise Book of Muscles 2e*. Lotus Publishing. Chichester, UK/North Atlantic Books, Berkeley, USA.

Jarmey, C.: 2006. *The Concise Book of the Moving Body*. Lotus Publishing. Chichester, UK/North Atlantic Books, Berkeley, USA.

Kendall, F.P., McCreary, E.K., Provance, P.G., Rodgers, M. & Romani, W.: 2010. *Muscle Testing and Function With Posture and Pain, 5e*. Lippincott, Williams and Wilkins, Baltimore, USA.

Lee, D.G. 2004: *The Pelvic Girdle: An Approach to the Examination and Treatment of the Lumbopelvic-Hip Region*. Churchill Livingstone, Edinburgh.

Martin, C.: 2002. *Functional Movement Development, 2e*. W. B. Saunders Co., London.

Richardson, C., Jull, G., Hodges, P. & Hides, J.: 1999. *Therapeutic Exercise for Spinal Segmental Stabilisation in Low Back Pain: Scientific Basis and Clinical Approach*. Churchill Livingstone, Edinburgh.

Thomas, C.L.: 1997. *Taber's Cyclopaedic Medical Dictionary, 18e*. FA Davis, Philadelphia, USA.

Wilmore, J.H. & Costill, D.L.: 1994. *Physiology of Sport & Exercise*. Human Kinetics, Champaign, USA.

Index

Patient Name:

POSTURAL ASSESSMENT SHEET – UPPER BODY

Muscles	Date:	Date:	Date:
Upper trapezius			
Levator scapulae			
Sternocleidomastoid			
Scalenes			
Latissimus dorsi			
Pectoralis major			
Pectoralis minor			
Coracoid muscles Biceps brachii short head Coracobrachialis			
Subscapularis			
Infraspinatus			

POSTURAL ASSESSMENT SHEET – LOWER BODY

Muscles	Date:	Date:	Date:
Gastrocnemius			
Soleus			
Medial hamstrings			
Lateral hamstrings			
Tensor fasciae latae / iliotibial band			
Adductors			
Rectus femoris			

POSTURAL ASSESSMENT SHEET – TRUNK / PELVIS AND HIP

Muscles	Date:	Date:	Date:
Piriformis			
Quadratus lumborum			
Psoas major and iliacus			
Lumbar spine erector spinae			

Key: E = Equal. L/R = Short on left or right side.

	1st	2nd	3rd	4th
Gluteus maximus	○	○	○	○
Hamstrings	○	○	○	○
Contralateral erector spinae	○	○	○	○
Ipsilateral erector spinae	○	○	○	○

Hip extension firing pattern – left side.

	1st	2nd	3rd	4th
Gluteus maximus	○	○	○	○
Hamstrings	○	○	○	○
Contralateral erector spinae	○	○	○	○
Ipsilateral erector spinae	○	○	○	○

Hip extension firing pattern – right side.

MUSCLE WEAKNESS ASSESSMENT SHEET

Muscles	Date:	Date:	Date:
Gluteus maximus			
Gluteus medius			
Posterior fibres of gluteus medius			
Serratus anterior			
Lower fibres of trapezius			

Key: E = Equal. L/R = Weakness on left or right side.

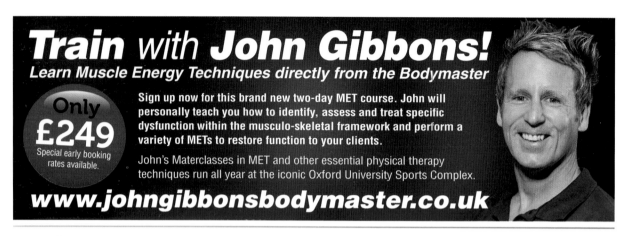
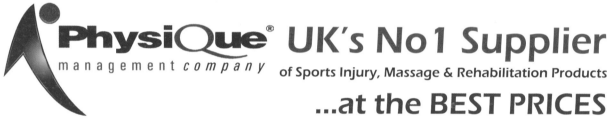
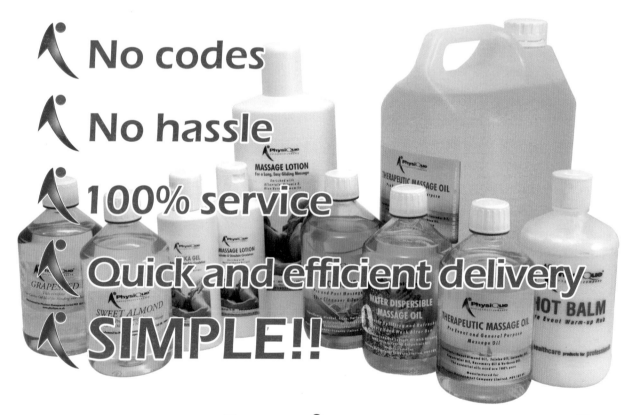